BLOOD GLUCOSE JOURNAL

This journal belongs to:

____

Disclaimer: This journal is ***not*** *intended to diagnose or treat anything. You should consult a doctor before using this journal. No liability will be accepted for any use or misuse. You use at your own risk and accept all liability.*

BLOOD GLUCOSE JOURNAL

BY VIVIAN TENORIO

JAV PUBLISHING

*Disclaimer: This journal is **not** intended to diagnose or treat anything. You should consult a doctor before using this journal. No liability will be accepted for any use or misuse. You use at your own risk and accept all liability.*

www.viviantenorio.com

ISBN-10: 0615786839

ISBN-13: 978-0615786834

"Happiness does not consist in pastimes and amusements but in virtuous activities." -Aristotle

MY DOCTOR

NAME: ____________________________________

PHONE: __________________________________

Disclaimer: This journal is ***not*** *intended to diagnose or treat anything. You should consult a doctor before using this journal. No liability will be accepted for any use or misuse. You use at your own risk and accept all liability.*

BLOOD GLUCOSE JOURNAL

Date: ____________________

	Before	After
BREAKFAST		

COMMENTS: (note exercise, illness, stress, special foods, or other factors that may affect your numbers.)

	Before	After
LUNCH		

COMMENTS: (note exercise, illness, stress, special foods, or other factors that may affect your numbers.)

	Before	After
DINNER		

COMMENTS: (note exercise, illness, stress, special foods, or other factors that may affect your numbers.)

	Before	After
NIGHT		

COMMENTS: (note exercise, illness, stress, special foods, or other factors that may affect your numbers.)

	Before	After
OTHER		

COMMENTS: (note exercise, illness, stress, special foods, or other factors that may affect your numbers.)

	Before	After
OTHER		

COMMENTS: (note exercise, illness, stress, special foods, or other factors that may affect your numbers.)

Date: ____________________

	Before	After
BREAKFAST		

COMMENTS: (note exercise, illness, stress, special foods, or other factors that may affect your numbers.)

	Before	After
LUNCH		

COMMENTS: (note exercise, illness, stress, special foods, or other factors that may affect your numbers.)

	Before	After
DINNER		

COMMENTS: (note exercise, illness, stress, special foods, or other factors that may affect your numbers.)

	Before	After
NIGHT		

COMMENTS: (note exercise, illness, stress, special foods, or other factors that may affect your numbers.)

	Before	After
OTHER		

COMMENTS: (note exercise, illness, stress, special foods, or other factors that may affect your numbers.)

	Before	After
OTHER		

COMMENTS: (note exercise, illness, stress, special foods, or other factors that may affect your numbers.)

BLOOD GLUCOSE JOURNAL

Date: ____________________

	Before	After
BREAKFAST		

COMMENTS: (note exercise, illness, stress, special foods, or other factors that may affect your numbers.)

	Before	After
LUNCH		

COMMENTS: (note exercise, illness, stress, special foods, or other factors that may affect your numbers.)

	Before	After
DINNER		

COMMENTS: (note exercise, illness, stress, special foods, or other factors that may affect your numbers.)

	Before	After
NIGHT		

COMMENTS: (note exercise, illness, stress, special foods, or other factors that may affect your numbers.)

	Before	After
OTHER		

COMMENTS: (note exercise, illness, stress, special foods, or other factors that may affect your numbers.)

	Before	After
OTHER		

COMMENTS: (note exercise, illness, stress, special foods, or other factors that may affect your numbers.)

Date: ____________________

	Before	After
BREAKFAST		

COMMENTS: (note exercise, illness, stress, special foods, or other factors that may affect your numbers.)

	Before	After
LUNCH		

COMMENTS: (note exercise, illness, stress, special foods, or other factors that may affect your numbers.)

	Before	After
DINNER		

COMMENTS: (note exercise, illness, stress, special foods, or other factors that may affect your numbers.)

	Before	After
NIGHT		

COMMENTS: (note exercise, illness, stress, special foods, or other factors that may affect your numbers.)

	Before	After
OTHER		

COMMENTS: (note exercise, illness, stress, special foods, or other factors that may affect your numbers.)

	Before	After
OTHER		

COMMENTS: (note exercise, illness, stress, special foods, or other factors that may affect your numbers.)

BLOOD GLUCOSE JOURNAL

Date: ___________________

	Before	After
BREAKFAST		

COMMENTS: (note exercise, illness, stress, special foods, or other factors that may affect your numbers.)

	Before	After
LUNCH		

COMMENTS: (note exercise, illness, stress, special foods, or other factors that may affect your numbers.)

	Before	After
DINNER		

COMMENTS: (note exercise, illness, stress, special foods, or other factors that may affect your numbers.)

	Before	After
NIGHT		

COMMENTS: (note exercise, illness, stress, special foods, or other factors that may affect your numbers.)

	Before	After
OTHER		

COMMENTS: (note exercise, illness, stress, special foods, or other factors that may affect your numbers.)

	Before	After
OTHER		

COMMENTS: (note exercise, illness, stress, special foods, or other factors that may affect your numbers.)

Date: ____________________

	Before	After
BREAKFAST		

COMMENTS: (note exercise, illness, stress, special foods, or other factors that may affect your numbers.)

	Before	After
LUNCH		

COMMENTS: (note exercise, illness, stress, special foods, or other factors that may affect your numbers.)

	Before	After
DINNER		

COMMENTS: (note exercise, illness, stress, special foods, or other factors that may affect your numbers.)

	Before	After
NIGHT		

COMMENTS: (note exercise, illness, stress, special foods, or other factors that may affect your numbers.)

	Before	After
OTHER		

COMMENTS: (note exercise, illness, stress, special foods, or other factors that may affect your numbers.)

	Before	After
OTHER		

COMMENTS: (note exercise, illness, stress, special foods, or other factors that may affect your numbers.)

BLOOD GLUCOSE JOURNAL

Date: ________________

	Before	After
BREAKFAST		

COMMENTS: (note exercise, illness, stress, special foods, or other factors that may affect your numbers.)

	Before	After
LUNCH		

COMMENTS: (note exercise, illness, stress, special foods, or other factors that may affect your numbers.)

	Before	After
DINNER		

COMMENTS: (note exercise, illness, stress, special foods, or other factors that may affect your numbers.)

	Before	After
NIGHT		

COMMENTS: (note exercise, illness, stress, special foods, or other factors that may affect your numbers.)

	Before	After
OTHER		

COMMENTS: (note exercise, illness, stress, special foods, or other factors that may affect your numbers.)

	Before	After
OTHER		

COMMENTS: (note exercise, illness, stress, special foods, or other factors that may affect your numbers.)

Date: ____________________

	Before	After
BREAKFAST		

COMMENTS: (note exercise, illness, stress, special foods, or other factors that may affect your numbers.)

	Before	After
LUNCH		

COMMENTS: (note exercise, illness, stress, special foods, or other factors that may affect your numbers.)

	Before	After
DINNER		

COMMENTS: (note exercise, illness, stress, special foods, or other factors that may affect your numbers.)

	Before	After
NIGHT		

COMMENTS: (note exercise, illness, stress, special foods, or other factors that may affect your numbers.)

	Before	After
OTHER		

COMMENTS: (note exercise, illness, stress, special foods, or other factors that may affect your numbers.)

	Before	After
OTHER		

COMMENTS: (note exercise, illness, stress, special foods, or other factors that may affect your numbers.)

BLOOD GLUCOSE JOURNAL

Date: ____________________

	Before	After
BREAKFAST		

COMMENTS: (note exercise, illness, stress, special foods, or other factors that may affect your numbers.)

	Before	After
LUNCH		

COMMENTS: (note exercise, illness, stress, special foods, or other factors that may affect your numbers.)

	Before	After
DINNER		

COMMENTS: (note exercise, illness, stress, special foods, or other factors that may affect your numbers.)

	Before	After
NIGHT		

COMMENTS: (note exercise, illness, stress, special foods, or other factors that may affect your numbers.)

	Before	After
OTHER		

COMMENTS: (note exercise, illness, stress, special foods, or other factors that may affect your numbers.)

	Before	After
OTHER		

COMMENTS: (note exercise, illness, stress, special foods, or other factors that may affect your numbers.)

Date: ___________________

	Before	After
BREAKFAST		

COMMENTS: (note exercise, illness, stress, special foods, or other factors that may affect your numbers.)

	Before	After
LUNCH		

COMMENTS: (note exercise, illness, stress, special foods, or other factors that may affect your numbers.)

	Before	After
DINNER		

COMMENTS: (note exercise, illness, stress, special foods, or other factors that may affect your numbers.)

	Before	After
NIGHT		

COMMENTS: (note exercise, illness, stress, special foods, or other factors that may affect your numbers.)

	Before	After
OTHER		

COMMENTS: (note exercise, illness, stress, special foods, or other factors that may affect your numbers.)

	Before	After
OTHER		

COMMENTS: (note exercise, illness, stress, special foods, or other factors that may affect your numbers.)

BLOOD GLUCOSE JOURNAL

Date: ___________________

	Before	After
BREAKFAST		

COMMENTS: (note exercise, illness, stress, special foods, or other factors that may affect your numbers.)

	Before	After
LUNCH		

COMMENTS: (note exercise, illness, stress, special foods, or other factors that may affect your numbers.)

	Before	After
DINNER		

COMMENTS: (note exercise, illness, stress, special foods, or other factors that may affect your numbers.)

	Before	After
NIGHT		

COMMENTS: (note exercise, illness, stress, special foods, or other factors that may affect your numbers.)

	Before	After
OTHER		

COMMENTS: (note exercise, illness, stress, special foods, or other factors that may affect your numbers.)

	Before	After
OTHER		

COMMENTS: (note exercise, illness, stress, special foods, or other factors that may affect your numbers.)

Date: ____________________

	Before	After
BREAKFAST		

COMMENTS: (note exercise, illness, stress, special foods, or other factors that may affect your numbers.)

	Before	After
LUNCH		

COMMENTS: (note exercise, illness, stress, special foods, or other factors that may affect your numbers.)

	Before	After
DINNER		

COMMENTS: (note exercise, illness, stress, special foods, or other factors that may affect your numbers.)

	Before	After
NIGHT		

COMMENTS: (note exercise, illness, stress, special foods, or other factors that may affect your numbers.)

	Before	After
OTHER		

COMMENTS: (note exercise, illness, stress, special foods, or other factors that may affect your numbers.)

	Before	After
OTHER		

COMMENTS: (note exercise, illness, stress, special foods, or other factors that may affect your numbers.)

BLOOD GLUCOSE JOURNAL

Date: ___________________

	Before	After
BREAKFAST		

COMMENTS: (note exercise, illness, stress, special foods, or other factors that may affect your numbers.)

	Before	After
LUNCH		

COMMENTS: (note exercise, illness, stress, special foods, or other factors that may affect your numbers.)

	Before	After
DINNER		

COMMENTS: (note exercise, illness, stress, special foods, or other factors that may affect your numbers.)

	Before	After
NIGHT		

COMMENTS: (note exercise, illness, stress, special foods, or other factors that may affect your numbers.)

	Before	After
OTHER		

COMMENTS: (note exercise, illness, stress, special foods, or other factors that may affect your numbers.)

	Before	After
OTHER		

COMMENTS: (note exercise, illness, stress, special foods, or other factors that may affect your numbers.)

Date: ___________________

	Before	After
BREAKFAST		

COMMENTS: (note exercise, illness, stress, special foods, or other factors that may affect your numbers.)

	Before	After
LUNCH		

COMMENTS: (note exercise, illness, stress, special foods, or other factors that may affect your numbers.)

	Before	After
DINNER		

COMMENTS: (note exercise, illness, stress, special foods, or other factors that may affect your numbers.)

	Before	After
NIGHT		

COMMENTS: (note exercise, illness, stress, special foods, or other factors that may affect your numbers.)

	Before	After
OTHER		

COMMENTS: (note exercise, illness, stress, special foods, or other factors that may affect your numbers.)

	Before	After
OTHER		

COMMENTS: (note exercise, illness, stress, special foods, or other factors that may affect your numbers.)

BLOOD GLUCOSE JOURNAL

Date: ___________________

	Before	After
BREAKFAST		

COMMENTS: (note exercise, illness, stress, special foods, or other factors that may affect your numbers.)

	Before	After
LUNCH		

COMMENTS: (note exercise, illness, stress, special foods, or other factors that may affect your numbers.)

	Before	After
DINNER		

COMMENTS: (note exercise, illness, stress, special foods, or other factors that may affect your numbers.)

	Before	After
NIGHT		

COMMENTS: (note exercise, illness, stress, special foods, or other factors that may affect your numbers.)

	Before	After
OTHER		

COMMENTS: (note exercise, illness, stress, special foods, or other factors that may affect your numbers.)

	Before	After
OTHER		

COMMENTS: (note exercise, illness, stress, special foods, or other factors that may affect your numbers.)

Date: ____________

	Before	After
BREAKFAST		

COMMENTS: (note exercise, illness, stress, special foods, or other factors that may affect your numbers.)

	Before	After
LUNCH		

COMMENTS: (note exercise, illness, stress, special foods, or other factors that may affect your numbers.)

	Before	After
DINNER		

COMMENTS: (note exercise, illness, stress, special foods, or other factors that may affect your numbers.)

	Before	After
NIGHT		

COMMENTS: (note exercise, illness, stress, special foods, or other factors that may affect your numbers.)

	Before	After
OTHER		

COMMENTS: (note exercise, illness, stress, special foods, or other factors that may affect your numbers.)

	Before	After
OTHER		

COMMENTS: (note exercise, illness, stress, special foods, or other factors that may affect your numbers.)

BLOOD GLUCOSE JOURNAL

Date: ____________________

	Before	After
BREAKFAST		

COMMENTS: (note exercise, illness, stress, special foods, or other factors that may affect your numbers.)

	Before	After
LUNCH		

COMMENTS: (note exercise, illness, stress, special foods, or other factors that may affect your numbers.)

	Before	After
DINNER		

COMMENTS: (note exercise, illness, stress, special foods, or other factors that may affect your numbers.)

	Before	After
NIGHT		

COMMENTS: (note exercise, illness, stress, special foods, or other factors that may affect your numbers.)

	Before	After
OTHER		

COMMENTS: (note exercise, illness, stress, special foods, or other factors that may affect your numbers.)

	Before	After
OTHER		

COMMENTS: (note exercise, illness, stress, special foods, or other factors that may affect your numbers.)

Date: ____________________

	Before	After
BREAKFAST		

COMMENTS: (note exercise, illness, stress, special foods, or other factors that may affect your numbers.)

	Before	After
LUNCH		

COMMENTS: (note exercise, illness, stress, special foods, or other factors that may affect your numbers.)

	Before	After
DINNER		

COMMENTS: (note exercise, illness, stress, special foods, or other factors that may affect your numbers.)

	Before	After
NIGHT		

COMMENTS: (note exercise, illness, stress, special foods, or other factors that may affect your numbers.)

	Before	After
OTHER		

COMMENTS: (note exercise, illness, stress, special foods, or other factors that may affect your numbers.)

	Before	After
OTHER		

COMMENTS: (note exercise, illness, stress, special foods, or other factors that may affect your numbers.)

BLOOD GLUCOSE JOURNAL

Date: ____________________

	Before	After
BREAKFAST		

COMMENTS: (note exercise, illness, stress, special foods, or other factors that may affect your numbers.)

	Before	After
LUNCH		

COMMENTS: (note exercise, illness, stress, special foods, or other factors that may affect your numbers.)

	Before	After
DINNER		

COMMENTS: (note exercise, illness, stress, special foods, or other factors that may affect your numbers.)

	Before	After
NIGHT		

COMMENTS: (note exercise, illness, stress, special foods, or other factors that may affect your numbers.)

	Before	After
OTHER		

COMMENTS: (note exercise, illness, stress, special foods, or other factors that may affect your numbers.)

	Before	After
OTHER		

COMMENTS: (note exercise, illness, stress, special foods, or other factors that may affect your numbers.)

Date: ________________

	Before	After
BREAKFAST		

COMMENTS: (note exercise, illness, stress, special foods, or other factors that may affect your numbers.)

	Before	After
LUNCH		

COMMENTS: (note exercise, illness, stress, special foods, or other factors that may affect your numbers.)

	Before	After
DINNER		

COMMENTS: (note exercise, illness, stress, special foods, or other factors that may affect your numbers.)

	Before	After
NIGHT		

COMMENTS: (note exercise, illness, stress, special foods, or other factors that may affect your numbers.)

	Before	After
OTHER		

COMMENTS: (note exercise, illness, stress, special foods, or other factors that may affect your numbers.)

	Before	After
OTHER		

COMMENTS: (note exercise, illness, stress, special foods, or other factors that may affect your numbers.)

BLOOD GLUCOSE JOURNAL

Date: ____________________

	Before	After
BREAKFAST		

COMMENTS: (note exercise, illness, stress, special foods, or other factors that may affect your numbers.)

	Before	After
LUNCH		

COMMENTS: (note exercise, illness, stress, special foods, or other factors that may affect your numbers.)

	Before	After
DINNER		

COMMENTS: (note exercise, illness, stress, special foods, or other factors that may affect your numbers.)

	Before	After
NIGHT		

COMMENTS: (note exercise, illness, stress, special foods, or other factors that may affect your numbers.)

	Before	After
OTHER		

COMMENTS: (note exercise, illness, stress, special foods, or other factors that may affect your numbers.)

	Before	After
OTHER		

COMMENTS: (note exercise, illness, stress, special foods, or other factors that may affect your numbers.)

Date: ____________________

	Before	After
BREAKFAST		

COMMENTS: (note exercise, illness, stress, special foods, or other factors that may affect your numbers.)

	Before	After
LUNCH		

COMMENTS: (note exercise, illness, stress, special foods, or other factors that may affect your numbers.)

	Before	After
DINNER		

COMMENTS: (note exercise, illness, stress, special foods, or other factors that may affect your numbers.)

	Before	After
NIGHT		

COMMENTS: (note exercise, illness, stress, special foods, or other factors that may affect your numbers.)

	Before	After
OTHER		

COMMENTS: (note exercise, illness, stress, special foods, or other factors that may affect your numbers.)

	Before	After
OTHER		

COMMENTS: (note exercise, illness, stress, special foods, or other factors that may affect your numbers.)

BLOOD GLUCOSE JOURNAL

Date: ____________________

	Before	After
BREAKFAST		

COMMENTS: (note exercise, illness, stress, special foods, or other factors that may affect your numbers.)

	Before	After
LUNCH		

COMMENTS: (note exercise, illness, stress, special foods, or other factors that may affect your numbers.)

	Before	After
DINNER		

COMMENTS: (note exercise, illness, stress, special foods, or other factors that may affect your numbers.)

	Before	After
NIGHT		

COMMENTS: (note exercise, illness, stress, special foods, or other factors that may affect your numbers.)

	Before	After
OTHER		

COMMENTS: (note exercise, illness, stress, special foods, or other factors that may affect your numbers.)

	Before	After
OTHER		

COMMENTS: (note exercise, illness, stress, special foods, or other factors that may affect your numbers.)

Date: ______________

	Before	After
BREAKFAST		

COMMENTS: (note exercise, illness, stress, special foods, or other factors that may affect your numbers.)

	Before	After
LUNCH		

COMMENTS: (note exercise, illness, stress, special foods, or other factors that may affect your numbers.)

	Before	After
DINNER		

COMMENTS: (note exercise, illness, stress, special foods, or other factors that may affect your numbers.)

	Before	After
NIGHT		

COMMENTS: (note exercise, illness, stress, special foods, or other factors that may affect your numbers.)

	Before	After
OTHER		

COMMENTS: (note exercise, illness, stress, special foods, or other factors that may affect your numbers.)

	Before	After
OTHER		

COMMENTS: (note exercise, illness, stress, special foods, or other factors that may affect your numbers.)

BLOOD GLUCOSE JOURNAL

Date: ____________________

	Before	After
BREAKFAST		

COMMENTS: (note exercise, illness, stress, special foods, or other factors that may affect your numbers.)

	Before	After
LUNCH		

COMMENTS: (note exercise, illness, stress, special foods, or other factors that may affect your numbers.)

	Before	After
DINNER		

COMMENTS: (note exercise, illness, stress, special foods, or other factors that may affect your numbers.)

	Before	After
NIGHT		

COMMENTS: (note exercise, illness, stress, special foods, or other factors that may affect your numbers.)

	Before	After
OTHER		

COMMENTS: (note exercise, illness, stress, special foods, or other factors that may affect your numbers.)

	Before	After
OTHER		

COMMENTS: (note exercise, illness, stress, special foods, or other factors that may affect your numbers.)

Date: ________________

	Before	After
BREAKFAST		

COMMENTS: (note exercise, illness, stress, special foods, or other factors that may affect your numbers.)

	Before	After
LUNCH		

COMMENTS: (note exercise, illness, stress, special foods, or other factors that may affect your numbers.)

	Before	After
DINNER		

COMMENTS: (note exercise, illness, stress, special foods, or other factors that may affect your numbers.)

	Before	After
NIGHT		

COMMENTS: (note exercise, illness, stress, special foods, or other factors that may affect your numbers.)

	Before	After
OTHER		

COMMENTS: (note exercise, illness, stress, special foods, or other factors that may affect your numbers.)

	Before	After
OTHER		

COMMENTS: (note exercise, illness, stress, special foods, or other factors that may affect your numbers.)

BLOOD GLUCOSE JOURNAL

Date: ____________________

	Before	After
BREAKFAST		

COMMENTS: (note exercise, illness, stress, special foods, or other factors that may affect your numbers.)

	Before	After
LUNCH		

COMMENTS: (note exercise, illness, stress, special foods, or other factors that may affect your numbers.)

	Before	After
DINNER		

COMMENTS: (note exercise, illness, stress, special foods, or other factors that may affect your numbers.)

	Before	After
NIGHT		

COMMENTS: (note exercise, illness, stress, special foods, or other factors that may affect your numbers.)

	Before	After
OTHER		

COMMENTS: (note exercise, illness, stress, special foods, or other factors that may affect your numbers.)

	Before	After
OTHER		

COMMENTS: (note exercise, illness, stress, special foods, or other factors that may affect your numbers.)

Date: ___________________

	Before	After
BREAKFAST		

COMMENTS: (note exercise, illness, stress, special foods, or other factors that may affect your numbers.)

	Before	After
LUNCH		

COMMENTS: (note exercise, illness, stress, special foods, or other factors that may affect your numbers.)

	Before	After
DINNER		

COMMENTS: (note exercise, illness, stress, special foods, or other factors that may affect your numbers.)

	Before	After
NIGHT		

COMMENTS: (note exercise, illness, stress, special foods, or other factors that may affect your numbers.)

	Before	After
OTHER		

COMMENTS: (note exercise, illness, stress, special foods, or other factors that may affect your numbers.)

	Before	After
OTHER		

COMMENTS: (note exercise, illness, stress, special foods, or other factors that may affect your numbers.)

BLOOD GLUCOSE JOURNAL

Date: ________________

	Before	After
BREAKFAST		

COMMENTS: (note exercise, illness, stress, special foods, or other factors that may affect your numbers.)

	Before	After
LUNCH		

COMMENTS: (note exercise, illness, stress, special foods, or other factors that may affect your numbers.)

	Before	After
DINNER		

COMMENTS: (note exercise, illness, stress, special foods, or other factors that may affect your numbers.)

	Before	After
NIGHT		

COMMENTS: (note exercise, illness, stress, special foods, or other factors that may affect your numbers.)

	Before	After
OTHER		

COMMENTS: (note exercise, illness, stress, special foods, or other factors that may affect your numbers.)

	Before	After
OTHER		

COMMENTS: (note exercise, illness, stress, special foods, or other factors that may affect your numbers.)

Date: ____________________

	Before	After
BREAKFAST		

COMMENTS: (note exercise, illness, stress, special foods, or other factors that may affect your numbers.)

	Before	After
LUNCH		

COMMENTS: (note exercise, illness, stress, special foods, or other factors that may affect your numbers.)

	Before	After
DINNER		

COMMENTS: (note exercise, illness, stress, special foods, or other factors that may affect your numbers.)

	Before	After
NIGHT		

COMMENTS: (note exercise, illness, stress, special foods, or other factors that may affect your numbers.)

	Before	After
OTHER		

COMMENTS: (note exercise, illness, stress, special foods, or other factors that may affect your numbers.)

	Before	After
OTHER		

COMMENTS: (note exercise, illness, stress, special foods, or other factors that may affect your numbers.)

BLOOD GLUCOSE JOURNAL

Date: ____________________

	Before	After
BREAKFAST		

COMMENTS: (note exercise, illness, stress, special foods, or other factors that may affect your numbers.)

	Before	After
LUNCH		

COMMENTS: (note exercise, illness, stress, special foods, or other factors that may affect your numbers.)

	Before	After
DINNER		

COMMENTS: (note exercise, illness, stress, special foods, or other factors that may affect your numbers.)

	Before	After
NIGHT		

COMMENTS: (note exercise, illness, stress, special foods, or other factors that may affect your numbers.)

	Before	After
OTHER		

COMMENTS: (note exercise, illness, stress, special foods, or other factors that may affect your numbers.)

	Before	After
OTHER		

COMMENTS: (note exercise, illness, stress, special foods, or other factors that may affect your numbers.)

Date: ___________________

	Before	After
BREAKFAST		

COMMENTS: (note exercise, illness, stress, special foods, or other factors that may affect your numbers.)

	Before	After
LUNCH		

COMMENTS: (note exercise, illness, stress, special foods, or other factors that may affect your numbers.)

	Before	After
DINNER		

COMMENTS: (note exercise, illness, stress, special foods, or other factors that may affect your numbers.)

	Before	After
NIGHT		

COMMENTS: (note exercise, illness, stress, special foods, or other factors that may affect your numbers.)

	Before	After
OTHER		

COMMENTS: (note exercise, illness, stress, special foods, or other factors that may affect your numbers.)

	Before	After
OTHER		

COMMENTS: (note exercise, illness, stress, special foods, or other factors that may affect your numbers.)

BLOOD GLUCOSE JOURNAL

Date: ____________________

	Before	After
BREAKFAST		

COMMENTS: (note exercise, illness, stress, special foods, or other factors that may affect your numbers.)

	Before	After
LUNCH		

COMMENTS: (note exercise, illness, stress, special foods, or other factors that may affect your numbers.)

	Before	After
DINNER		

COMMENTS: (note exercise, illness, stress, special foods, or other factors that may affect your numbers.)

	Before	After
NIGHT		

COMMENTS: (note exercise, illness, stress, special foods, or other factors that may affect your numbers.)

	Before	After
OTHER		

COMMENTS: (note exercise, illness, stress, special foods, or other factors that may affect your numbers.)

	Before	After
OTHER		

COMMENTS: (note exercise, illness, stress, special foods, or other factors that may affect your numbers.)

Date: ___________________

	Before	After
BREAKFAST		

COMMENTS: (note exercise, illness, stress, special foods, or other factors that may affect your numbers.)

	Before	After
LUNCH		

COMMENTS: (note exercise, illness, stress, special foods, or other factors that may affect your numbers.)

	Before	After
DINNER		

COMMENTS: (note exercise, illness, stress, special foods, or other factors that may affect your numbers.)

	Before	After
NIGHT		

COMMENTS: (note exercise, illness, stress, special foods, or other factors that may affect your numbers.)

	Before	After
OTHER		

COMMENTS: (note exercise, illness, stress, special foods, or other factors that may affect your numbers.)

	Before	After
OTHER		

COMMENTS: (note exercise, illness, stress, special foods, or other factors that may affect your numbers.)

BLOOD GLUCOSE JOURNAL

Date: ____________________

	Before	After
BREAKFAST		

COMMENTS: (note exercise, illness, stress, special foods, or other factors that may affect your numbers.)

	Before	After
LUNCH		

COMMENTS: (note exercise, illness, stress, special foods, or other factors that may affect your numbers.)

	Before	After
DINNER		

COMMENTS: (note exercise, illness, stress, special foods, or other factors that may affect your numbers.)

	Before	After
NIGHT		

COMMENTS: (note exercise, illness, stress, special foods, or other factors that may affect your numbers.)

	Before	After
OTHER		

COMMENTS: (note exercise, illness, stress, special foods, or other factors that may affect your numbers.)

	Before	After
OTHER		

COMMENTS: (note exercise, illness, stress, special foods, or other factors that may affect your numbers.)

Date: ____________________

	Before	After
BREAKFAST		

COMMENTS: (note exercise, illness, stress, special foods, or other factors that may affect your numbers.)

	Before	After
LUNCH		

COMMENTS: (note exercise, illness, stress, special foods, or other factors that may affect your numbers.)

	Before	After
DINNER		

COMMENTS: (note exercise, illness, stress, special foods, or other factors that may affect your numbers.)

	Before	After
NIGHT		

COMMENTS: (note exercise, illness, stress, special foods, or other factors that may affect your numbers.)

	Before	After
OTHER		

COMMENTS: (note exercise, illness, stress, special foods, or other factors that may affect your numbers.)

	Before	After
OTHER		

COMMENTS: (note exercise, illness, stress, special foods, or other factors that may affect your numbers.)

BLOOD GLUCOSE JOURNAL

Date: ____________________

	Before	After
BREAKFAST		

COMMENTS: (note exercise, illness, stress, special foods, or other factors that may affect your numbers.)

	Before	After
LUNCH		

COMMENTS: (note exercise, illness, stress, special foods, or other factors that may affect your numbers.)

	Before	After
DINNER		

COMMENTS: (note exercise, illness, stress, special foods, or other factors that may affect your numbers.)

	Before	After
NIGHT		

COMMENTS: (note exercise, illness, stress, special foods, or other factors that may affect your numbers.)

	Before	After
OTHER		

COMMENTS: (note exercise, illness, stress, special foods, or other factors that may affect your numbers.)

	Before	After
OTHER		

COMMENTS: (note exercise, illness, stress, special foods, or other factors that may affect your numbers.)

Date: ____________________

	Before	After
BREAKFAST		

COMMENTS: (note exercise, illness, stress, special foods, or other factors that may affect your numbers.)

	Before	After
LUNCH		

COMMENTS: (note exercise, illness, stress, special foods, or other factors that may affect your numbers.)

	Before	After
DINNER		

COMMENTS: (note exercise, illness, stress, special foods, or other factors that may affect your numbers.)

	Before	After
NIGHT		

COMMENTS: (note exercise, illness, stress, special foods, or other factors that may affect your numbers.)

	Before	After
OTHER		

COMMENTS: (note exercise, illness, stress, special foods, or other factors that may affect your numbers.)

	Before	After
OTHER		

COMMENTS: (note exercise, illness, stress, special foods, or other factors that may affect your numbers.)

BLOOD GLUCOSE JOURNAL

Date: ____________________

	Before	After
BREAKFAST		

COMMENTS: (note exercise, illness, stress, special foods, or other factors that may affect your numbers.)

	Before	After
LUNCH		

COMMENTS: (note exercise, illness, stress, special foods, or other factors that may affect your numbers.)

	Before	After
DINNER		

COMMENTS: (note exercise, illness, stress, special foods, or other factors that may affect your numbers.)

	Before	After
NIGHT		

COMMENTS: (note exercise, illness, stress, special foods, or other factors that may affect your numbers.)

	Before	After
OTHER		

COMMENTS: (note exercise, illness, stress, special foods, or other factors that may affect your numbers.)

	Before	After
OTHER		

COMMENTS: (note exercise, illness, stress, special foods, or other factors that may affect your numbers.)

Date: ____________________

	Before	After
BREAKFAST		

COMMENTS: (note exercise, illness, stress, special foods, or other factors that may affect your numbers.)

	Before	After
LUNCH		

COMMENTS: (note exercise, illness, stress, special foods, or other factors that may affect your numbers.)

	Before	After
DINNER		

COMMENTS: (note exercise, illness, stress, special foods, or other factors that may affect your numbers.)

	Before	After
NIGHT		

COMMENTS: (note exercise, illness, stress, special foods, or other factors that may affect your numbers.)

	Before	After
OTHER		

COMMENTS: (note exercise, illness, stress, special foods, or other factors that may affect your numbers.)

	Before	After
OTHER		

COMMENTS: (note exercise, illness, stress, special foods, or other factors that may affect your numbers.)

BLOOD GLUCOSE JOURNAL

Date: ____________________

	Before	After
BREAKFAST		

COMMENTS: (note exercise, illness, stress, special foods, or other factors that may affect your numbers.)

	Before	After
LUNCH		

COMMENTS: (note exercise, illness, stress, special foods, or other factors that may affect your numbers.)

	Before	After
DINNER		

COMMENTS: (note exercise, illness, stress, special foods, or other factors that may affect your numbers.)

	Before	After
NIGHT		

COMMENTS: (note exercise, illness, stress, special foods, or other factors that may affect your numbers.)

	Before	After
OTHER		

COMMENTS: (note exercise, illness, stress, special foods, or other factors that may affect your numbers.)

	Before	After
OTHER		

COMMENTS: (note exercise, illness, stress, special foods, or other factors that may affect your numbers.)

Date: ________________

	Before	After
BREAKFAST		

COMMENTS: (note exercise, illness, stress, special foods, or other factors that may affect your numbers.)

	Before	After
LUNCH		

COMMENTS: (note exercise, illness, stress, special foods, or other factors that may affect your numbers.)

	Before	After
DINNER		

COMMENTS: (note exercise, illness, stress, special foods, or other factors that may affect your numbers.)

	Before	After
NIGHT		

COMMENTS: (note exercise, illness, stress, special foods, or other factors that may affect your numbers.)

	Before	After
OTHER		

COMMENTS: (note exercise, illness, stress, special foods, or other factors that may affect your numbers.)

	Before	After
OTHER		

COMMENTS: (note exercise, illness, stress, special foods, or other factors that may affect your numbers.)

BLOOD GLUCOSE JOURNAL

Date: ____________________

	Before	After
BREAKFAST		

COMMENTS: (note exercise, illness, stress, special foods, or other factors that may affect your numbers.)

	Before	After
LUNCH		

COMMENTS: (note exercise, illness, stress, special foods, or other factors that may affect your numbers.)

	Before	After
DINNER		

COMMENTS: (note exercise, illness, stress, special foods, or other factors that may affect your numbers.)

	Before	After
NIGHT		

COMMENTS: (note exercise, illness, stress, special foods, or other factors that may affect your numbers.)

	Before	After
OTHER		

COMMENTS: (note exercise, illness, stress, special foods, or other factors that may affect your numbers.)

	Before	After
OTHER		

COMMENTS: (note exercise, illness, stress, special foods, or other factors that may affect your numbers.)

Date: ________________

	Before	After
BREAKFAST		

COMMENTS: (note exercise, illness, stress, special foods, or other factors that may affect your numbers.)

	Before	After
LUNCH		

COMMENTS: (note exercise, illness, stress, special foods, or other factors that may affect your numbers.)

	Before	After
DINNER		

COMMENTS: (note exercise, illness, stress, special foods, or other factors that may affect your numbers.)

	Before	After
NIGHT		

COMMENTS: (note exercise, illness, stress, special foods, or other factors that may affect your numbers.)

	Before	After
OTHER		

COMMENTS: (note exercise, illness, stress, special foods, or other factors that may affect your numbers.)

	Before	After
OTHER		

COMMENTS: (note exercise, illness, stress, special foods, or other factors that may affect your numbers.)

BLOOD GLUCOSE JOURNAL

Date: ________________

	Before	After
BREAKFAST		

COMMENTS: (note exercise, illness, stress, special foods, or other factors that may affect your numbers.)

	Before	After
LUNCH		

COMMENTS: (note exercise, illness, stress, special foods, or other factors that may affect your numbers.)

	Before	After
DINNER		

COMMENTS: (note exercise, illness, stress, special foods, or other factors that may affect your numbers.)

	Before	After
NIGHT		

COMMENTS: (note exercise, illness, stress, special foods, or other factors that may affect your numbers.)

	Before	After
OTHER		

COMMENTS: (note exercise, illness, stress, special foods, or other factors that may affect your numbers.)

	Before	After
OTHER		

COMMENTS: (note exercise, illness, stress, special foods, or other factors that may affect your numbers.)

Date: ____________________

	Before	After
BREAKFAST		

COMMENTS: (note exercise, illness, stress, special foods, or other factors that may affect your numbers.)

	Before	After
LUNCH		

COMMENTS: (note exercise, illness, stress, special foods, or other factors that may affect your numbers.)

	Before	After
DINNER		

COMMENTS: (note exercise, illness, stress, special foods, or other factors that may affect your numbers.)

	Before	After
NIGHT		

COMMENTS: (note exercise, illness, stress, special foods, or other factors that may affect your numbers.)

	Before	After
OTHER		

COMMENTS: (note exercise, illness, stress, special foods, or other factors that may affect your numbers.)

	Before	After
OTHER		

COMMENTS: (note exercise, illness, stress, special foods, or other factors that may affect your numbers.)

BLOOD GLUCOSE JOURNAL

Date: ____________________

	Before	After
BREAKFAST		

COMMENTS: (note exercise, illness, stress, special foods, or other factors that may affect your numbers.)

	Before	After
LUNCH		

COMMENTS: (note exercise, illness, stress, special foods, or other factors that may affect your numbers.)

	Before	After
DINNER		

COMMENTS: (note exercise, illness, stress, special foods, or other factors that may affect your numbers.)

	Before	After
NIGHT		

COMMENTS: (note exercise, illness, stress, special foods, or other factors that may affect your numbers.)

	Before	After
OTHER		

COMMENTS: (note exercise, illness, stress, special foods, or other factors that may affect your numbers.)

	Before	After
OTHER		

COMMENTS: (note exercise, illness, stress, special foods, or other factors that may affect your numbers.)

Date: ____________________

	Before	After
BREAKFAST		

COMMENTS: (note exercise, illness, stress, special foods, or other factors that may affect your numbers.)

	Before	After
LUNCH		

COMMENTS: (note exercise, illness, stress, special foods, or other factors that may affect your numbers.)

	Before	After
DINNER		

COMMENTS: (note exercise, illness, stress, special foods, or other factors that may affect your numbers.)

	Before	After
NIGHT		

COMMENTS: (note exercise, illness, stress, special foods, or other factors that may affect your numbers.)

	Before	After
OTHER		

COMMENTS: (note exercise, illness, stress, special foods, or other factors that may affect your numbers.)

	Before	After
OTHER		

COMMENTS: (note exercise, illness, stress, special foods, or other factors that may affect your numbers.)

BLOOD GLUCOSE JOURNAL

Date: ___________________

	Before	After
BREAKFAST		

COMMENTS: (note exercise, illness, stress, special foods, or other factors that may affect your numbers.)

	Before	After
LUNCH		

COMMENTS: (note exercise, illness, stress, special foods, or other factors that may affect your numbers.)

	Before	After
DINNER		

COMMENTS: (note exercise, illness, stress, special foods, or other factors that may affect your numbers.)

	Before	After
NIGHT		

COMMENTS: (note exercise, illness, stress, special foods, or other factors that may affect your numbers.)

	Before	After
OTHER		

COMMENTS: (note exercise, illness, stress, special foods, or other factors that may affect your numbers.)

	Before	After
OTHER		

COMMENTS: (note exercise, illness, stress, special foods, or other factors that may affect your numbers.)

Date: ________________

	Before	After
BREAKFAST		

COMMENTS: (note exercise, illness, stress, special foods, or other factors that may affect your numbers.)

	Before	After
LUNCH		

COMMENTS: (note exercise, illness, stress, special foods, or other factors that may affect your numbers.)

	Before	After
DINNER		

COMMENTS: (note exercise, illness, stress, special foods, or other factors that may affect your numbers.)

	Before	After
NIGHT		

COMMENTS: (note exercise, illness, stress, special foods, or other factors that may affect your numbers.)

	Before	After
OTHER		

COMMENTS: (note exercise, illness, stress, special foods, or other factors that may affect your numbers.)

	Before	After
OTHER		

COMMENTS: (note exercise, illness, stress, special foods, or other factors that may affect your numbers.)

BLOOD GLUCOSE JOURNAL

Date: ____________________

	Before	After
BREAKFAST		

COMMENTS: (note exercise, illness, stress, special foods, or other factors that may affect your numbers.)

	Before	After
LUNCH		

COMMENTS: (note exercise, illness, stress, special foods, or other factors that may affect your numbers.)

	Before	After
DINNER		

COMMENTS: (note exercise, illness, stress, special foods, or other factors that may affect your numbers.)

	Before	After
NIGHT		

COMMENTS: (note exercise, illness, stress, special foods, or other factors that may affect your numbers.)

	Before	After
OTHER		

COMMENTS: (note exercise, illness, stress, special foods, or other factors that may affect your numbers.)

	Before	After
OTHER		

COMMENTS: (note exercise, illness, stress, special foods, or other factors that may affect your numbers.)

Date: ________________

	Before	After
BREAKFAST		

COMMENTS: (note exercise, illness, stress, special foods, or other factors that may affect your numbers.)

	Before	After
LUNCH		

COMMENTS: (note exercise, illness, stress, special foods, or other factors that may affect your numbers.)

	Before	After
DINNER		

COMMENTS: (note exercise, illness, stress, special foods, or other factors that may affect your numbers.)

	Before	After
NIGHT		

COMMENTS: (note exercise, illness, stress, special foods, or other factors that may affect your numbers.)

	Before	After
OTHER		

COMMENTS: (note exercise, illness, stress, special foods, or other factors that may affect your numbers.)

	Before	After
OTHER		

COMMENTS: (note exercise, illness, stress, special foods, or other factors that may affect your numbers.)

BLOOD GLUCOSE JOURNAL

Date: ____________________

	Before	After
BREAKFAST		

COMMENTS: (note exercise, illness, stress, special foods, or other factors that may affect your numbers.)

	Before	After
LUNCH		

COMMENTS: (note exercise, illness, stress, special foods, or other factors that may affect your numbers.)

	Before	After
DINNER		

COMMENTS: (note exercise, illness, stress, special foods, or other factors that may affect your numbers.)

	Before	After
NIGHT		

COMMENTS: (note exercise, illness, stress, special foods, or other factors that may affect your numbers.)

	Before	After
OTHER		

COMMENTS: (note exercise, illness, stress, special foods, or other factors that may affect your numbers.)

	Before	After
OTHER		

COMMENTS: (note exercise, illness, stress, special foods, or other factors that may affect your numbers.)

Date: ____________________

	Before	After
BREAKFAST		

COMMENTS: (note exercise, illness, stress, special foods, or other factors that may affect your numbers.)

	Before	After
LUNCH		

COMMENTS: (note exercise, illness, stress, special foods, or other factors that may affect your numbers.)

	Before	After
DINNER		

COMMENTS: (note exercise, illness, stress, special foods, or other factors that may affect your numbers.)

	Before	After
NIGHT		

COMMENTS: (note exercise, illness, stress, special foods, or other factors that may affect your numbers.)

	Before	After
OTHER		

COMMENTS: (note exercise, illness, stress, special foods, or other factors that may affect your numbers.)

	Before	After
OTHER		

COMMENTS: (note exercise, illness, stress, special foods, or other factors that may affect your numbers.)

BLOOD GLUCOSE JOURNAL

Date: ____________________

	Before	After
BREAKFAST		

COMMENTS: (note exercise, illness, stress, special foods, or other factors that may affect your numbers.)

	Before	After
LUNCH		

COMMENTS: (note exercise, illness, stress, special foods, or other factors that may affect your numbers.)

	Before	After
DINNER		

COMMENTS: (note exercise, illness, stress, special foods, or other factors that may affect your numbers.)

	Before	After
NIGHT		

COMMENTS: (note exercise, illness, stress, special foods, or other factors that may affect your numbers.)

	Before	After
OTHER		

COMMENTS: (note exercise, illness, stress, special foods, or other factors that may affect your numbers.)

	Before	After
OTHER		

COMMENTS: (note exercise, illness, stress, special foods, or other factors that may affect your numbers.)

Date: ____________________

	Before	After
BREAKFAST		

COMMENTS: (note exercise, illness, stress, special foods, or other factors that may affect your numbers.)

	Before	After
LUNCH		

COMMENTS: (note exercise, illness, stress, special foods, or other factors that may affect your numbers.)

	Before	After
DINNER		

COMMENTS: (note exercise, illness, stress, special foods, or other factors that may affect your numbers.)

	Before	After
NIGHT		

COMMENTS: (note exercise, illness, stress, special foods, or other factors that may affect your numbers.)

	Before	After
OTHER		

COMMENTS: (note exercise, illness, stress, special foods, or other factors that may affect your numbers.)

	Before	After
OTHER		

COMMENTS: (note exercise, illness, stress, special foods, or other factors that may affect your numbers.)

BLOOD GLUCOSE JOURNAL

Date: ________________

	Before	After
BREAKFAST		

COMMENTS: (note exercise, illness, stress, special foods, or other factors that may affect your numbers.)

	Before	After
LUNCH		

COMMENTS: (note exercise, illness, stress, special foods, or other factors that may affect your numbers.)

	Before	After
DINNER		

COMMENTS: (note exercise, illness, stress, special foods, or other factors that may affect your numbers.)

	Before	After
NIGHT		

COMMENTS: (note exercise, illness, stress, special foods, or other factors that may affect your numbers.)

	Before	After
OTHER		

COMMENTS: (note exercise, illness, stress, special foods, or other factors that may affect your numbers.)

	Before	After
OTHER		

COMMENTS: (note exercise, illness, stress, special foods, or other factors that may affect your numbers.)

Date: ________________

	Before	After
BREAKFAST		

COMMENTS: (note exercise, illness, stress, special foods, or other factors that may affect your numbers.)

	Before	After
LUNCH		

COMMENTS: (note exercise, illness, stress, special foods, or other factors that may affect your numbers.)

	Before	After
DINNER		

COMMENTS: (note exercise, illness, stress, special foods, or other factors that may affect your numbers.)

	Before	After
NIGHT		

COMMENTS: (note exercise, illness, stress, special foods, or other factors that may affect your numbers.)

	Before	After
OTHER		

COMMENTS: (note exercise, illness, stress, special foods, or other factors that may affect your numbers.)

	Before	After
OTHER		

COMMENTS: (note exercise, illness, stress, special foods, or other factors that may affect your numbers.)

BLOOD GLUCOSE JOURNAL

Date: ___________________

	Before	After
BREAKFAST		

COMMENTS: (note exercise, illness, stress, special foods, or other factors that may affect your numbers.)

	Before	After
LUNCH		

COMMENTS: (note exercise, illness, stress, special foods, or other factors that may affect your numbers.)

	Before	After
DINNER		

COMMENTS: (note exercise, illness, stress, special foods, or other factors that may affect your numbers.)

	Before	After
NIGHT		

COMMENTS: (note exercise, illness, stress, special foods, or other factors that may affect your numbers.)

	Before	After
OTHER		

COMMENTS: (note exercise, illness, stress, special foods, or other factors that may affect your numbers.)

	Before	After
OTHER		

COMMENTS: (note exercise, illness, stress, special foods, or other factors that may affect your numbers.)

Date: ____________________

	Before	After
BREAKFAST		

COMMENTS: (note exercise, illness, stress, special foods, or other factors that may affect your numbers.)

	Before	After
LUNCH		

COMMENTS: (note exercise, illness, stress, special foods, or other factors that may affect your numbers.)

	Before	After
DINNER		

COMMENTS: (note exercise, illness, stress, special foods, or other factors that may affect your numbers.)

	Before	After
NIGHT		

COMMENTS: (note exercise, illness, stress, special foods, or other factors that may affect your numbers.)

	Before	After
OTHER		

COMMENTS: (note exercise, illness, stress, special foods, or other factors that may affect your numbers.)

	Before	After
OTHER		

COMMENTS: (note exercise, illness, stress, special foods, or other factors that may affect your numbers.)

BLOOD GLUCOSE JOURNAL

Date: ____________________

	Before	After
BREAKFAST		

COMMENTS: (note exercise, illness, stress, special foods, or other factors that may affect your numbers.)

	Before	After
LUNCH		

COMMENTS: (note exercise, illness, stress, special foods, or other factors that may affect your numbers.)

	Before	After
DINNER		

COMMENTS: (note exercise, illness, stress, special foods, or other factors that may affect your numbers.)

	Before	After
NIGHT		

COMMENTS: (note exercise, illness, stress, special foods, or other factors that may affect your numbers.)

	Before	After
OTHER		

COMMENTS: (note exercise, illness, stress, special foods, or other factors that may affect your numbers.)

	Before	After
OTHER		

COMMENTS: (note exercise, illness, stress, special foods, or other factors that may affect your numbers.)

Date: ________________

	Before	After
BREAKFAST		

COMMENTS: (note exercise, illness, stress, special foods, or other factors that may affect your numbers.)

	Before	After
LUNCH		

COMMENTS: (note exercise, illness, stress, special foods, or other factors that may affect your numbers.)

	Before	After
DINNER		

COMMENTS: (note exercise, illness, stress, special foods, or other factors that may affect your numbers.)

	Before	After
NIGHT		

COMMENTS: (note exercise, illness, stress, special foods, or other factors that may affect your numbers.)

	Before	After
OTHER		

COMMENTS: (note exercise, illness, stress, special foods, or other factors that may affect your numbers.)

	Before	After
OTHER		

COMMENTS: (note exercise, illness, stress, special foods, or other factors that may affect your numbers.)

BLOOD GLUCOSE JOURNAL

Date: ________________

	Before	After
BREAKFAST		

COMMENTS: (note exercise, illness, stress, special foods, or other factors that may affect your numbers.)

	Before	After
LUNCH		

COMMENTS: (note exercise, illness, stress, special foods, or other factors that may affect your numbers.)

	Before	After
DINNER		

COMMENTS: (note exercise, illness, stress, special foods, or other factors that may affect your numbers.)

	Before	After
NIGHT		

COMMENTS: (note exercise, illness, stress, special foods, or other factors that may affect your numbers.)

	Before	After
OTHER		

COMMENTS: (note exercise, illness, stress, special foods, or other factors that may affect your numbers.)

	Before	After
OTHER		

COMMENTS: (note exercise, illness, stress, special foods, or other factors that may affect your numbers.)

Date: ____________________

	Before	After
BREAKFAST		

COMMENTS: (note exercise, illness, stress, special foods, or other factors that may affect your numbers.)

	Before	After
LUNCH		

COMMENTS: (note exercise, illness, stress, special foods, or other factors that may affect your numbers.)

	Before	After
DINNER		

COMMENTS: (note exercise, illness, stress, special foods, or other factors that may affect your numbers.)

	Before	After
NIGHT		

COMMENTS: (note exercise, illness, stress, special foods, or other factors that may affect your numbers.)

	Before	After
OTHER		

COMMENTS: (note exercise, illness, stress, special foods, or other factors that may affect your numbers.)

	Before	After
OTHER		

COMMENTS: (note exercise, illness, stress, special foods, or other factors that may affect your numbers.)

BLOOD GLUCOSE JOURNAL

Date: ____________________

	Before	After
BREAKFAST		

COMMENTS: (note exercise, illness, stress, special foods, or other factors that may affect your numbers.)

	Before	After
LUNCH		

COMMENTS: (note exercise, illness, stress, special foods, or other factors that may affect your numbers.)

	Before	After
DINNER		

COMMENTS: (note exercise, illness, stress, special foods, or other factors that may affect your numbers.)

	Before	After
NIGHT		

COMMENTS: (note exercise, illness, stress, special foods, or other factors that may affect your numbers.)

	Before	After
OTHER		

COMMENTS: (note exercise, illness, stress, special foods, or other factors that may affect your numbers.)

	Before	After
OTHER		

COMMENTS: (note exercise, illness, stress, special foods, or other factors that may affect your numbers.)

Date: ____________________

	Before	After
BREAKFAST		

COMMENTS: (note exercise, illness, stress, special foods, or other factors that may affect your numbers.)

	Before	After
LUNCH		

COMMENTS: (note exercise, illness, stress, special foods, or other factors that may affect your numbers.)

	Before	After
DINNER		

COMMENTS: (note exercise, illness, stress, special foods, or other factors that may affect your numbers.)

	Before	After
NIGHT		

COMMENTS: (note exercise, illness, stress, special foods, or other factors that may affect your numbers.)

	Before	After
OTHER		

COMMENTS: (note exercise, illness, stress, special foods, or other factors that may affect your numbers.)

	Before	After
OTHER		

COMMENTS: (note exercise, illness, stress, special foods, or other factors that may affect your numbers.)

BLOOD GLUCOSE JOURNAL

Date: ____________________

	Before	After
BREAKFAST		

COMMENTS: (note exercise, illness, stress, special foods, or other factors that may affect your numbers.)

	Before	After
LUNCH		

COMMENTS: (note exercise, illness, stress, special foods, or other factors that may affect your numbers.)

	Before	After
DINNER		

COMMENTS: (note exercise, illness, stress, special foods, or other factors that may affect your numbers.)

	Before	After
NIGHT		

COMMENTS: (note exercise, illness, stress, special foods, or other factors that may affect your numbers.)

	Before	After
OTHER		

COMMENTS: (note exercise, illness, stress, special foods, or other factors that may affect your numbers.)

	Before	After
OTHER		

COMMENTS: (note exercise, illness, stress, special foods, or other factors that may affect your numbers.)

Date: ____________________

	Before	After
BREAKFAST		

COMMENTS: (note exercise, illness, stress, special foods, or other factors that may affect your numbers.)

	Before	After
LUNCH		

COMMENTS: (note exercise, illness, stress, special foods, or other factors that may affect your numbers.)

	Before	After
DINNER		

COMMENTS: (note exercise, illness, stress, special foods, or other factors that may affect your numbers.)

	Before	After
NIGHT		

COMMENTS: (note exercise, illness, stress, special foods, or other factors that may affect your numbers.)

	Before	After
OTHER		

COMMENTS: (note exercise, illness, stress, special foods, or other factors that may affect your numbers.)

	Before	After
OTHER		

COMMENTS: (note exercise, illness, stress, special foods, or other factors that may affect your numbers.)

BLOOD GLUCOSE JOURNAL

Date: ____________________

	Before	After
BREAKFAST		

COMMENTS: (note exercise, illness, stress, special foods, or other factors that may affect your numbers.)

	Before	After
LUNCH		

COMMENTS: (note exercise, illness, stress, special foods, or other factors that may affect your numbers.)

	Before	After
DINNER		

COMMENTS: (note exercise, illness, stress, special foods, or other factors that may affect your numbers.)

	Before	After
NIGHT		

COMMENTS: (note exercise, illness, stress, special foods, or other factors that may affect your numbers.)

	Before	After
OTHER		

COMMENTS: (note exercise, illness, stress, special foods, or other factors that may affect your numbers.)

	Before	After
OTHER		

COMMENTS: (note exercise, illness, stress, special foods, or other factors that may affect your numbers.)

Date: ___________________

	Before	After
BREAKFAST		

COMMENTS: (note exercise, illness, stress, special foods, or other factors that may affect your numbers.)

	Before	After
LUNCH		

COMMENTS: (note exercise, illness, stress, special foods, or other factors that may affect your numbers.)

	Before	After
DINNER		

COMMENTS: (note exercise, illness, stress, special foods, or other factors that may affect your numbers.)

	Before	After
NIGHT		

COMMENTS: (note exercise, illness, stress, special foods, or other factors that may affect your numbers.)

	Before	After
OTHER		

COMMENTS: (note exercise, illness, stress, special foods, or other factors that may affect your numbers.)

	Before	After
OTHER		

COMMENTS: (note exercise, illness, stress, special foods, or other factors that may affect your numbers.)

BLOOD GLUCOSE JOURNAL

Date: ____________________

	Before	After
BREAKFAST		

COMMENTS: (note exercise, illness, stress, special foods, or other factors that may affect your numbers.)

	Before	After
LUNCH		

COMMENTS: (note exercise, illness, stress, special foods, or other factors that may affect your numbers.)

	Before	After
DINNER		

COMMENTS: (note exercise, illness, stress, special foods, or other factors that may affect your numbers.)

	Before	After
NIGHT		

COMMENTS: (note exercise, illness, stress, special foods, or other factors that may affect your numbers.)

	Before	After
OTHER		

COMMENTS: (note exercise, illness, stress, special foods, or other factors that may affect your numbers.)

	Before	After
OTHER		

COMMENTS: (note exercise, illness, stress, special foods, or other factors that may affect your numbers.)

Date: ____________________

	Before	After
BREAKFAST		

COMMENTS: (note exercise, illness, stress, special foods, or other factors that may affect your numbers.)

	Before	After
LUNCH		

COMMENTS: (note exercise, illness, stress, special foods, or other factors that may affect your numbers.)

	Before	After
DINNER		

COMMENTS: (note exercise, illness, stress, special foods, or other factors that may affect your numbers.)

	Before	After
NIGHT		

COMMENTS: (note exercise, illness, stress, special foods, or other factors that may affect your numbers.)

	Before	After
OTHER		

COMMENTS: (note exercise, illness, stress, special foods, or other factors that may affect your numbers.)

	Before	After
OTHER		

COMMENTS: (note exercise, illness, stress, special foods, or other factors that may affect your numbers.)

BLOOD GLUCOSE JOURNAL

Date: ____________________

	Before	After
BREAKFAST		

COMMENTS: (note exercise, illness, stress, special foods, or other factors that may affect your numbers.)

	Before	After
LUNCH		

COMMENTS: (note exercise, illness, stress, special foods, or other factors that may affect your numbers.)

	Before	After
DINNER		

COMMENTS: (note exercise, illness, stress, special foods, or other factors that may affect your numbers.)

	Before	After
NIGHT		

COMMENTS: (note exercise, illness, stress, special foods, or other factors that may affect your numbers.)

	Before	After
OTHER		

COMMENTS: (note exercise, illness, stress, special foods, or other factors that may affect your numbers.)

	Before	After
OTHER		

COMMENTS: (note exercise, illness, stress, special foods, or other factors that may affect your numbers.)

Date: ___________________

	Before	After
BREAKFAST		

COMMENTS: (note exercise, illness, stress, special foods, or other factors that may affect your numbers.)

	Before	After
LUNCH		

COMMENTS: (note exercise, illness, stress, special foods, or other factors that may affect your numbers.)

	Before	After
DINNER		

COMMENTS: (note exercise, illness, stress, special foods, or other factors that may affect your numbers.)

	Before	After
NIGHT		

COMMENTS: (note exercise, illness, stress, special foods, or other factors that may affect your numbers.)

	Before	After
OTHER		

COMMENTS: (note exercise, illness, stress, special foods, or other factors that may affect your numbers.)

	Before	After
OTHER		

COMMENTS: (note exercise, illness, stress, special foods, or other factors that may affect your numbers.)

BLOOD GLUCOSE JOURNAL

Date: ____________________

	Before	After
BREAKFAST		

COMMENTS: (note exercise, illness, stress, special foods, or other factors that may affect your numbers.)

	Before	After
LUNCH		

COMMENTS: (note exercise, illness, stress, special foods, or other factors that may affect your numbers.)

	Before	After
DINNER		

COMMENTS: (note exercise, illness, stress, special foods, or other factors that may affect your numbers.)

	Before	After
NIGHT		

COMMENTS: (note exercise, illness, stress, special foods, or other factors that may affect your numbers.)

	Before	After
OTHER		

COMMENTS: (note exercise, illness, stress, special foods, or other factors that may affect your numbers.)

	Before	After
OTHER		

COMMENTS: (note exercise, illness, stress, special foods, or other factors that may affect your numbers.)

Date: ________________

	Before	After
BREAKFAST		

COMMENTS: (note exercise, illness, stress, special foods, or other factors that may affect your numbers.)

	Before	After
LUNCH		

COMMENTS: (note exercise, illness, stress, special foods, or other factors that may affect your numbers.)

	Before	After
DINNER		

COMMENTS: (note exercise, illness, stress, special foods, or other factors that may affect your numbers.)

	Before	After
NIGHT		

COMMENTS: (note exercise, illness, stress, special foods, or other factors that may affect your numbers.)

	Before	After
OTHER		

COMMENTS: (note exercise, illness, stress, special foods, or other factors that may affect your numbers.)

	Before	After
OTHER		

COMMENTS: (note exercise, illness, stress, special foods, or other factors that may affect your numbers.)

BLOOD GLUCOSE JOURNAL

Date: ____________________

	Before	After
BREAKFAST		

COMMENTS: (note exercise, illness, stress, special foods, or other factors that may affect your numbers.)

	Before	After
LUNCH		

COMMENTS: (note exercise, illness, stress, special foods, or other factors that may affect your numbers.)

	Before	After
DINNER		

COMMENTS: (note exercise, illness, stress, special foods, or other factors that may affect your numbers.)

	Before	After
NIGHT		

COMMENTS: (note exercise, illness, stress, special foods, or other factors that may affect your numbers.)

	Before	After
OTHER		

COMMENTS: (note exercise, illness, stress, special foods, or other factors that may affect your numbers.)

	Before	After
OTHER		

COMMENTS: (note exercise, illness, stress, special foods, or other factors that may affect your numbers.)

Date: ___________________

	Before	After
BREAKFAST		

COMMENTS: (note exercise, illness, stress, special foods, or other factors that may affect your numbers.)

	Before	After
LUNCH		

COMMENTS: (note exercise, illness, stress, special foods, or other factors that may affect your numbers.)

	Before	After
DINNER		

COMMENTS: (note exercise, illness, stress, special foods, or other factors that may affect your numbers.)

	Before	After
NIGHT		

COMMENTS: (note exercise, illness, stress, special foods, or other factors that may affect your numbers.)

	Before	After
OTHER		

COMMENTS: (note exercise, illness, stress, special foods, or other factors that may affect your numbers.)

	Before	After
OTHER		

COMMENTS: (note exercise, illness, stress, special foods, or other factors that may affect your numbers.)

BLOOD GLUCOSE JOURNAL

Date: ____________________

	Before	After
BREAKFAST		

COMMENTS: (note exercise, illness, stress, special foods, or other factors that may affect your numbers.)

	Before	After
LUNCH		

COMMENTS: (note exercise, illness, stress, special foods, or other factors that may affect your numbers.)

	Before	After
DINNER		

COMMENTS: (note exercise, illness, stress, special foods, or other factors that may affect your numbers.)

	Before	After
NIGHT		

COMMENTS: (note exercise, illness, stress, special foods, or other factors that may affect your numbers.)

	Before	After
OTHER		

COMMENTS: (note exercise, illness, stress, special foods, or other factors that may affect your numbers.)

	Before	After
OTHER		

COMMENTS: (note exercise, illness, stress, special foods, or other factors that may affect your numbers.)

Date: ________________

	Before	After
BREAKFAST		

COMMENTS: (note exercise, illness, stress, special foods, or other factors that may affect your numbers.)

	Before	After
LUNCH		

COMMENTS: (note exercise, illness, stress, special foods, or other factors that may affect your numbers.)

	Before	After
DINNER		

COMMENTS: (note exercise, illness, stress, special foods, or other factors that may affect your numbers.)

	Before	After
NIGHT		

COMMENTS: (note exercise, illness, stress, special foods, or other factors that may affect your numbers.)

	Before	After
OTHER		

COMMENTS: (note exercise, illness, stress, special foods, or other factors that may affect your numbers.)

	Before	After
OTHER		

COMMENTS: (note exercise, illness, stress, special foods, or other factors that may affect your numbers.)

BLOOD GLUCOSE JOURNAL

Date: ___________________

	Before	After
BREAKFAST		

COMMENTS: (note exercise, illness, stress, special foods, or other factors that may affect your numbers.)

	Before	After
LUNCH		

COMMENTS: (note exercise, illness, stress, special foods, or other factors that may affect your numbers.)

	Before	After
DINNER		

COMMENTS: (note exercise, illness, stress, special foods, or other factors that may affect your numbers.)

	Before	After
NIGHT		

COMMENTS: (note exercise, illness, stress, special foods, or other factors that may affect your numbers.)

	Before	After
OTHER		

COMMENTS: (note exercise, illness, stress, special foods, or other factors that may affect your numbers.)

	Before	After
OTHER		

COMMENTS: (note exercise, illness, stress, special foods, or other factors that may affect your numbers.)

Date: ____________________

	Before	After
BREAKFAST		

COMMENTS: (note exercise, illness, stress, special foods, or other factors that may affect your numbers.)

	Before	After
LUNCH		

COMMENTS: (note exercise, illness, stress, special foods, or other factors that may affect your numbers.)

	Before	After
DINNER		

COMMENTS: (note exercise, illness, stress, special foods, or other factors that may affect your numbers.)

	Before	After
NIGHT		

COMMENTS: (note exercise, illness, stress, special foods, or other factors that may affect your numbers.)

	Before	After
OTHER		

COMMENTS: (note exercise, illness, stress, special foods, or other factors that may affect your numbers.)

	Before	After
OTHER		

COMMENTS: (note exercise, illness, stress, special foods, or other factors that may affect your numbers.)

BLOOD GLUCOSE JOURNAL

Date: ________________

	Before	After
BREAKFAST		

COMMENTS: (note exercise, illness, stress, special foods, or other factors that may affect your numbers.)

	Before	After
LUNCH		

COMMENTS: (note exercise, illness, stress, special foods, or other factors that may affect your numbers.)

	Before	After
DINNER		

COMMENTS: (note exercise, illness, stress, special foods, or other factors that may affect your numbers.)

	Before	After
NIGHT		

COMMENTS: (note exercise, illness, stress, special foods, or other factors that may affect your numbers.)

	Before	After
OTHER		

COMMENTS: (note exercise, illness, stress, special foods, or other factors that may affect your numbers.)

	Before	After
OTHER		

COMMENTS: (note exercise, illness, stress, special foods, or other factors that may affect your numbers.)

Date: ____________________

	Before	After
BREAKFAST		

COMMENTS: (note exercise, illness, stress, special foods, or other factors that may affect your numbers.)

	Before	After
LUNCH		

COMMENTS: (note exercise, illness, stress, special foods, or other factors that may affect your numbers.)

	Before	After
DINNER		

COMMENTS: (note exercise, illness, stress, special foods, or other factors that may affect your numbers.)

	Before	After
NIGHT		

COMMENTS: (note exercise, illness, stress, special foods, or other factors that may affect your numbers.)

	Before	After
OTHER		

COMMENTS: (note exercise, illness, stress, special foods, or other factors that may affect your numbers.)

	Before	After
OTHER		

COMMENTS: (note exercise, illness, stress, special foods, or other factors that may affect your numbers.)

BLOOD GLUCOSE JOURNAL

Date: ____________________

	Before	After
BREAKFAST		

COMMENTS: (note exercise, illness, stress, special foods, or other factors that may affect your numbers.)

	Before	After
LUNCH		

COMMENTS: (note exercise, illness, stress, special foods, or other factors that may affect your numbers.)

	Before	After
DINNER		

COMMENTS: (note exercise, illness, stress, special foods, or other factors that may affect your numbers.)

	Before	After
NIGHT		

COMMENTS: (note exercise, illness, stress, special foods, or other factors that may affect your numbers.)

	Before	After
OTHER		

COMMENTS: (note exercise, illness, stress, special foods, or other factors that may affect your numbers.)

	Before	After
OTHER		

COMMENTS: (note exercise, illness, stress, special foods, or other factors that may affect your numbers.)

Date: ____________

	Before	After
BREAKFAST		

COMMENTS: (note exercise, illness, stress, special foods, or other factors that may affect your numbers.)

	Before	After
LUNCH		

COMMENTS: (note exercise, illness, stress, special foods, or other factors that may affect your numbers.)

	Before	After
DINNER		

COMMENTS: (note exercise, illness, stress, special foods, or other factors that may affect your numbers.)

	Before	After
NIGHT		

COMMENTS: (note exercise, illness, stress, special foods, or other factors that may affect your numbers.)

	Before	After
OTHER		

COMMENTS: (note exercise, illness, stress, special foods, or other factors that may affect your numbers.)

	Before	After
OTHER		

COMMENTS: (note exercise, illness, stress, special foods, or other factors that may affect your numbers.)

BLOOD GLUCOSE JOURNAL

Date: ________________

	Before	After
BREAKFAST		

COMMENTS: (note exercise, illness, stress, special foods, or other factors that may affect your numbers.)

	Before	After
LUNCH		

COMMENTS: (note exercise, illness, stress, special foods, or other factors that may affect your numbers.)

	Before	After
DINNER		

COMMENTS: (note exercise, illness, stress, special foods, or other factors that may affect your numbers.)

	Before	After
NIGHT		

COMMENTS: (note exercise, illness, stress, special foods, or other factors that may affect your numbers.)

	Before	After
OTHER		

COMMENTS: (note exercise, illness, stress, special foods, or other factors that may affect your numbers.)

	Before	After
OTHER		

COMMENTS: (note exercise, illness, stress, special foods, or other factors that may affect your numbers.)

Date: ____________________

	Before	After
BREAKFAST		

COMMENTS: (note exercise, illness, stress, special foods, or other factors that may affect your numbers.)

	Before	After
LUNCH		

COMMENTS: (note exercise, illness, stress, special foods, or other factors that may affect your numbers.)

	Before	After
DINNER		

COMMENTS: (note exercise, illness, stress, special foods, or other factors that may affect your numbers.)

	Before	After
NIGHT		

COMMENTS: (note exercise, illness, stress, special foods, or other factors that may affect your numbers.)

	Before	After
OTHER		

COMMENTS: (note exercise, illness, stress, special foods, or other factors that may affect your numbers.)

	Before	After
OTHER		

COMMENTS: (note exercise, illness, stress, special foods, or other factors that may affect your numbers.)

BLOOD GLUCOSE JOURNAL

Date: ____________________

	Before	After
BREAKFAST		

COMMENTS: (note exercise, illness, stress, special foods, or other factors that may affect your numbers.)

	Before	After
LUNCH		

COMMENTS: (note exercise, illness, stress, special foods, or other factors that may affect your numbers.)

	Before	After
DINNER		

COMMENTS: (note exercise, illness, stress, special foods, or other factors that may affect your numbers.)

	Before	After
NIGHT		

COMMENTS: (note exercise, illness, stress, special foods, or other factors that may affect your numbers.)

	Before	After
OTHER		

COMMENTS: (note exercise, illness, stress, special foods, or other factors that may affect your numbers.)

	Before	After
OTHER		

COMMENTS: (note exercise, illness, stress, special foods, or other factors that may affect your numbers.)

Date: ________________

	Before	After
BREAKFAST		

COMMENTS: (note exercise, illness, stress, special foods, or other factors that may affect your numbers.)

	Before	After
LUNCH		

COMMENTS: (note exercise, illness, stress, special foods, or other factors that may affect your numbers.)

	Before	After
DINNER		

COMMENTS: (note exercise, illness, stress, special foods, or other factors that may affect your numbers.)

	Before	After
NIGHT		

COMMENTS: (note exercise, illness, stress, special foods, or other factors that may affect your numbers.)

	Before	After
OTHER		

COMMENTS: (note exercise, illness, stress, special foods, or other factors that may affect your numbers.)

	Before	After
OTHER		

COMMENTS: (note exercise, illness, stress, special foods, or other factors that may affect your numbers.)

BLOOD GLUCOSE JOURNAL

Date: ____________________

	Before	After
BREAKFAST		

COMMENTS: (note exercise, illness, stress, special foods, or other factors that may affect your numbers.)

	Before	After
LUNCH		

COMMENTS: (note exercise, illness, stress, special foods, or other factors that may affect your numbers.)

	Before	After
DINNER		

COMMENTS: (note exercise, illness, stress, special foods, or other factors that may affect your numbers.)

	Before	After
NIGHT		

COMMENTS: (note exercise, illness, stress, special foods, or other factors that may affect your numbers.)

	Before	After
OTHER		

COMMENTS: (note exercise, illness, stress, special foods, or other factors that may affect your numbers.)

	Before	After
OTHER		

COMMENTS: (note exercise, illness, stress, special foods, or other factors that may affect your numbers.)

Date: ____________________

	Before	After
BREAKFAST		

COMMENTS: (note exercise, illness, stress, special foods, or other factors that may affect your numbers.)

	Before	After
LUNCH		

COMMENTS: (note exercise, illness, stress, special foods, or other factors that may affect your numbers.)

	Before	After
DINNER		

COMMENTS: (note exercise, illness, stress, special foods, or other factors that may affect your numbers.)

	Before	After
NIGHT		

COMMENTS: (note exercise, illness, stress, special foods, or other factors that may affect your numbers.)

	Before	After
OTHER		

COMMENTS: (note exercise, illness, stress, special foods, or other factors that may affect your numbers.)

	Before	After
OTHER		

COMMENTS: (note exercise, illness, stress, special foods, or other factors that may affect your numbers.)

BLOOD GLUCOSE JOURNAL

Date: ____________________

	Before	After
BREAKFAST		

COMMENTS: (note exercise, illness, stress, special foods, or other factors that may affect your numbers.)

	Before	After
LUNCH		

COMMENTS: (note exercise, illness, stress, special foods, or other factors that may affect your numbers.)

	Before	After
DINNER		

COMMENTS: (note exercise, illness, stress, special foods, or other factors that may affect your numbers.)

	Before	After
NIGHT		

COMMENTS: (note exercise, illness, stress, special foods, or other factors that may affect your numbers.)

	Before	After
OTHER		

COMMENTS: (note exercise, illness, stress, special foods, or other factors that may affect your numbers.)

	Before	After
OTHER		

COMMENTS: (note exercise, illness, stress, special foods, or other factors that may affect your numbers.)

Date: ____________________

	Before	After
BREAKFAST		

COMMENTS: (note exercise, illness, stress, special foods, or other factors that may affect your numbers.)

	Before	After
LUNCH		

COMMENTS: (note exercise, illness, stress, special foods, or other factors that may affect your numbers.)

	Before	After
DINNER		

COMMENTS: (note exercise, illness, stress, special foods, or other factors that may affect your numbers.)

	Before	After
NIGHT		

COMMENTS: (note exercise, illness, stress, special foods, or other factors that may affect your numbers.)

	Before	After
OTHER		

COMMENTS: (note exercise, illness, stress, special foods, or other factors that may affect your numbers.)

	Before	After
OTHER		

COMMENTS: (note exercise, illness, stress, special foods, or other factors that may affect your numbers.)

BLOOD GLUCOSE JOURNAL

Date: ___________________

	Before	After
BREAKFAST		

COMMENTS: (note exercise, illness, stress, special foods, or other factors that may affect your numbers.)

	Before	After
LUNCH		

COMMENTS: (note exercise, illness, stress, special foods, or other factors that may affect your numbers.)

	Before	After
DINNER		

COMMENTS: (note exercise, illness, stress, special foods, or other factors that may affect your numbers.)

	Before	After
NIGHT		

COMMENTS: (note exercise, illness, stress, special foods, or other factors that may affect your numbers.)

	Before	After
OTHER		

COMMENTS: (note exercise, illness, stress, special foods, or other factors that may affect your numbers.)

	Before	After
OTHER		

COMMENTS: (note exercise, illness, stress, special foods, or other factors that may affect your numbers.)

Date: ____________________

	Before	After
BREAKFAST		

COMMENTS: (note exercise, illness, stress, special foods, or other factors that may affect your numbers.)

	Before	After
LUNCH		

COMMENTS: (note exercise, illness, stress, special foods, or other factors that may affect your numbers.)

	Before	After
DINNER		

COMMENTS: (note exercise, illness, stress, special foods, or other factors that may affect your numbers.)

	Before	After
NIGHT		

COMMENTS: (note exercise, illness, stress, special foods, or other factors that may affect your numbers.)

	Before	After
OTHER		

COMMENTS: (note exercise, illness, stress, special foods, or other factors that may affect your numbers.)

	Before	After
OTHER		

COMMENTS: (note exercise, illness, stress, special foods, or other factors that may affect your numbers.)

BLOOD GLUCOSE JOURNAL

Date: ____________________

	Before	After
BREAKFAST		

COMMENTS: (note exercise, illness, stress, special foods, or other factors that may affect your numbers.)

	Before	After
LUNCH		

COMMENTS: (note exercise, illness, stress, special foods, or other factors that may affect your numbers.)

	Before	After
DINNER		

COMMENTS: (note exercise, illness, stress, special foods, or other factors that may affect your numbers.)

	Before	After
NIGHT		

COMMENTS: (note exercise, illness, stress, special foods, or other factors that may affect your numbers.)

	Before	After
OTHER		

COMMENTS: (note exercise, illness, stress, special foods, or other factors that may affect your numbers.)

	Before	After
OTHER		

COMMENTS: (note exercise, illness, stress, special foods, or other factors that may affect your numbers.)

Date: ____________________

BREAKFAST	Before	After

COMMENTS: (note exercise, illness, stress, special foods, or other factors that may affect your numbers.)

LUNCH	Before	After

COMMENTS: (note exercise, illness, stress, special foods, or other factors that may affect your numbers.)

DINNER	Before	After

COMMENTS: (note exercise, illness, stress, special foods, or other factors that may affect your numbers.)

NIGHT	Before	After

COMMENTS: (note exercise, illness, stress, special foods, or other factors that may affect your numbers.)

OTHER	Before	After

COMMENTS: (note exercise, illness, stress, special foods, or other factors that may affect your numbers.)

OTHER	Before	After

COMMENTS: (note exercise, illness, stress, special foods, or other factors that may affect your numbers.)

BLOOD GLUCOSE JOURNAL

Date: ____________________

	Before	After
BREAKFAST		

COMMENTS: (note exercise, illness, stress, special foods, or other factors that may affect your numbers.)

	Before	After
LUNCH		

COMMENTS: (note exercise, illness, stress, special foods, or other factors that may affect your numbers.)

	Before	After
DINNER		

COMMENTS: (note exercise, illness, stress, special foods, or other factors that may affect your numbers.)

	Before	After
NIGHT		

COMMENTS: (note exercise, illness, stress, special foods, or other factors that may affect your numbers.)

	Before	After
OTHER		

COMMENTS: (note exercise, illness, stress, special foods, or other factors that may affect your numbers.)

	Before	After
OTHER		

COMMENTS: (note exercise, illness, stress, special foods, or other factors that may affect your numbers.)

Date: ____________________

	Before	After
BREAKFAST		

COMMENTS: (note exercise, illness, stress, special foods, or other factors that may affect your numbers.)

	Before	After
LUNCH		

COMMENTS: (note exercise, illness, stress, special foods, or other factors that may affect your numbers.)

	Before	After
DINNER		

COMMENTS: (note exercise, illness, stress, special foods, or other factors that may affect your numbers.)

	Before	After
NIGHT		

COMMENTS: (note exercise, illness, stress, special foods, or other factors that may affect your numbers.)

	Before	After
OTHER		

COMMENTS: (note exercise, illness, stress, special foods, or other factors that may affect your numbers.)

	Before	After
OTHER		

COMMENTS: (note exercise, illness, stress, special foods, or other factors that may affect your numbers.)

BLOOD GLUCOSE JOURNAL

Date: ________________

	Before	After
BREAKFAST		

COMMENTS: (note exercise, illness, stress, special foods, or other factors that may affect your numbers.)

	Before	After
LUNCH		

COMMENTS: (note exercise, illness, stress, special foods, or other factors that may affect your numbers.)

	Before	After
DINNER		

COMMENTS: (note exercise, illness, stress, special foods, or other factors that may affect your numbers.)

	Before	After
NIGHT		

COMMENTS: (note exercise, illness, stress, special foods, or other factors that may affect your numbers.)

	Before	After
OTHER		

COMMENTS: (note exercise, illness, stress, special foods, or other factors that may affect your numbers.)

	Before	After
OTHER		

COMMENTS: (note exercise, illness, stress, special foods, or other factors that may affect your numbers.)

Date: ____________________

	Before	After
BREAKFAST		

COMMENTS: (note exercise, illness, stress, special foods, or other factors that may affect your numbers.)

	Before	After
LUNCH		

COMMENTS: (note exercise, illness, stress, special foods, or other factors that may affect your numbers.)

	Before	After
DINNER		

COMMENTS: (note exercise, illness, stress, special foods, or other factors that may affect your numbers.)

	Before	After
NIGHT		

COMMENTS: (note exercise, illness, stress, special foods, or other factors that may affect your numbers.)

	Before	After
OTHER		

COMMENTS: (note exercise, illness, stress, special foods, or other factors that may affect your numbers.)

	Before	After
OTHER		

COMMENTS: (note exercise, illness, stress, special foods, or other factors that may affect your numbers.)

BLOOD GLUCOSE JOURNAL

Date: ____________________

	Before	After
BREAKFAST		

COMMENTS: (note exercise, illness, stress, special foods, or other factors that may affect your numbers.)

	Before	After
LUNCH		

COMMENTS: (note exercise, illness, stress, special foods, or other factors that may affect your numbers.)

	Before	After
DINNER		

COMMENTS: (note exercise, illness, stress, special foods, or other factors that may affect your numbers.)

	Before	After
NIGHT		

COMMENTS: (note exercise, illness, stress, special foods, or other factors that may affect your numbers.)

	Before	After
OTHER		

COMMENTS: (note exercise, illness, stress, special foods, or other factors that may affect your numbers.)

	Before	After
OTHER		

COMMENTS: (note exercise, illness, stress, special foods, or other factors that may affect your numbers.)

Date: ____________________

BREAKFAST	Before	After

COMMENTS: (note exercise, illness, stress, special foods, or other factors that may affect your numbers.)

LUNCH	Before	After

COMMENTS: (note exercise, illness, stress, special foods, or other factors that may affect your numbers.)

DINNER	Before	After

COMMENTS: (note exercise, illness, stress, special foods, or other factors that may affect your numbers.)

NIGHT	Before	After

COMMENTS: (note exercise, illness, stress, special foods, or other factors that may affect your numbers.)

OTHER	Before	After

COMMENTS: (note exercise, illness, stress, special foods, or other factors that may affect your numbers.)

OTHER	Before	After

COMMENTS: (note exercise, illness, stress, special foods, or other factors that may affect your numbers.)

BLOOD GLUCOSE JOURNAL

Date: ___________________

	Before	After
BREAKFAST		

COMMENTS: (note exercise, illness, stress, special foods, or other factors that may affect your numbers.)

	Before	After
LUNCH		

COMMENTS: (note exercise, illness, stress, special foods, or other factors that may affect your numbers.)

	Before	After
DINNER		

COMMENTS: (note exercise, illness, stress, special foods, or other factors that may affect your numbers.)

	Before	After
NIGHT		

COMMENTS: (note exercise, illness, stress, special foods, or other factors that may affect your numbers.)

	Before	After
OTHER		

COMMENTS: (note exercise, illness, stress, special foods, or other factors that may affect your numbers.)

	Before	After
OTHER		

COMMENTS: (note exercise, illness, stress, special foods, or other factors that may affect your numbers.)

Date: ____________________

	Before	After
BREAKFAST		

COMMENTS: (note exercise, illness, stress, special foods, or other factors that may affect your numbers.)

	Before	After
LUNCH		

COMMENTS: (note exercise, illness, stress, special foods, or other factors that may affect your numbers.)

	Before	After
DINNER		

COMMENTS: (note exercise, illness, stress, special foods, or other factors that may affect your numbers.)

	Before	After
NIGHT		

COMMENTS: (note exercise, illness, stress, special foods, or other factors that may affect your numbers.)

	Before	After
OTHER		

COMMENTS: (note exercise, illness, stress, special foods, or other factors that may affect your numbers.)

	Before	After
OTHER		

COMMENTS: (note exercise, illness, stress, special foods, or other factors that may affect your numbers.)

BLOOD GLUCOSE JOURNAL

Date: ____________________

	Before	After
BREAKFAST		

COMMENTS: (note exercise, illness, stress, special foods, or other factors that may affect your numbers.)

	Before	After
LUNCH		

COMMENTS: (note exercise, illness, stress, special foods, or other factors that may affect your numbers.)

	Before	After
DINNER		

COMMENTS: (note exercise, illness, stress, special foods, or other factors that may affect your numbers.)

	Before	After
NIGHT		

COMMENTS: (note exercise, illness, stress, special foods, or other factors that may affect your numbers.)

	Before	After
OTHER		

COMMENTS: (note exercise, illness, stress, special foods, or other factors that may affect your numbers.)

	Before	After
OTHER		

COMMENTS: (note exercise, illness, stress, special foods, or other factors that may affect your numbers.)

Date: ________________

	Before	After
BREAKFAST		

COMMENTS: (note exercise, illness, stress, special foods, or other factors that may affect your numbers.)

	Before	After
LUNCH		

COMMENTS: (note exercise, illness, stress, special foods, or other factors that may affect your numbers.)

	Before	After
DINNER		

COMMENTS: (note exercise, illness, stress, special foods, or other factors that may affect your numbers.)

	Before	After
NIGHT		

COMMENTS: (note exercise, illness, stress, special foods, or other factors that may affect your numbers.)

	Before	After
OTHER		

COMMENTS: (note exercise, illness, stress, special foods, or other factors that may affect your numbers.)

	Before	After
OTHER		

COMMENTS: (note exercise, illness, stress, special foods, or other factors that may affect your numbers.)

BLOOD GLUCOSE JOURNAL

Date: ____________________

	Before	After
BREAKFAST		

COMMENTS: (note exercise, illness, stress, special foods, or other factors that may affect your numbers.)

	Before	After
LUNCH		

COMMENTS: (note exercise, illness, stress, special foods, or other factors that may affect your numbers.)

	Before	After
DINNER		

COMMENTS: (note exercise, illness, stress, special foods, or other factors that may affect your numbers.)

	Before	After
NIGHT		

COMMENTS: (note exercise, illness, stress, special foods, or other factors that may affect your numbers.)

	Before	After
OTHER		

COMMENTS: (note exercise, illness, stress, special foods, or other factors that may affect your numbers.)

	Before	After
OTHER		

COMMENTS: (note exercise, illness, stress, special foods, or other factors that may affect your numbers.)

Date: ____________________

	Before	After
BREAKFAST		

COMMENTS: (note exercise, illness, stress, special foods, or other factors that may affect your numbers.)

	Before	After
LUNCH		

COMMENTS: (note exercise, illness, stress, special foods, or other factors that may affect your numbers.)

	Before	After
DINNER		

COMMENTS: (note exercise, illness, stress, special foods, or other factors that may affect your numbers.)

	Before	After
NIGHT		

COMMENTS: (note exercise, illness, stress, special foods, or other factors that may affect your numbers.)

	Before	After
OTHER		

COMMENTS: (note exercise, illness, stress, special foods, or other factors that may affect your numbers.)

	Before	After
OTHER		

COMMENTS: (note exercise, illness, stress, special foods, or other factors that may affect your numbers.)

BLOOD GLUCOSE JOURNAL

Date: ____________________

	Before	After
BREAKFAST		

COMMENTS: (note exercise, illness, stress, special foods, or other factors that may affect your numbers.)

	Before	After
LUNCH		

COMMENTS: (note exercise, illness, stress, special foods, or other factors that may affect your numbers.)

	Before	After
DINNER		

COMMENTS: (note exercise, illness, stress, special foods, or other factors that may affect your numbers.)

	Before	After
NIGHT		

COMMENTS: (note exercise, illness, stress, special foods, or other factors that may affect your numbers.)

	Before	After
OTHER		

COMMENTS: (note exercise, illness, stress, special foods, or other factors that may affect your numbers.)

	Before	After
OTHER		

COMMENTS: (note exercise, illness, stress, special foods, or other factors that may affect your numbers.)

Date: ___________________

	Before	After
BREAKFAST		

COMMENTS: (note exercise, illness, stress, special foods, or other factors that may affect your numbers.)

	Before	After
LUNCH		

COMMENTS: (note exercise, illness, stress, special foods, or other factors that may affect your numbers.)

	Before	After
DINNER		

COMMENTS: (note exercise, illness, stress, special foods, or other factors that may affect your numbers.)

	Before	After
NIGHT		

COMMENTS: (note exercise, illness, stress, special foods, or other factors that may affect your numbers.)

	Before	After
OTHER		

COMMENTS: (note exercise, illness, stress, special foods, or other factors that may affect your numbers.)

	Before	After
OTHER		

COMMENTS: (note exercise, illness, stress, special foods, or other factors that may affect your numbers.)

BLOOD GLUCOSE JOURNAL

Date: ____________________

	Before	After
BREAKFAST		

COMMENTS: (note exercise, illness, stress, special foods, or other factors that may affect your numbers.)

	Before	After
LUNCH		

COMMENTS: (note exercise, illness, stress, special foods, or other factors that may affect your numbers.)

	Before	After
DINNER		

COMMENTS: (note exercise, illness, stress, special foods, or other factors that may affect your numbers.)

	Before	After
NIGHT		

COMMENTS: (note exercise, illness, stress, special foods, or other factors that may affect your numbers.)

	Before	After
OTHER		

COMMENTS: (note exercise, illness, stress, special foods, or other factors that may affect your numbers.)

	Before	After
OTHER		

COMMENTS: (note exercise, illness, stress, special foods, or other factors that may affect your numbers.)

Date: ____________________

	Before	After
BREAKFAST		

COMMENTS: (note exercise, illness, stress, special foods, or other factors that may affect your numbers.)

	Before	After
LUNCH		

COMMENTS: (note exercise, illness, stress, special foods, or other factors that may affect your numbers.)

	Before	After
DINNER		

COMMENTS: (note exercise, illness, stress, special foods, or other factors that may affect your numbers.)

	Before	After
NIGHT		

COMMENTS: (note exercise, illness, stress, special foods, or other factors that may affect your numbers.)

	Before	After
OTHER		

COMMENTS: (note exercise, illness, stress, special foods, or other factors that may affect your numbers.)

	Before	After
OTHER		

COMMENTS: (note exercise, illness, stress, special foods, or other factors that may affect your numbers.)

BLOOD GLUCOSE JOURNAL

Date: ____________________

	Before	After
BREAKFAST		

COMMENTS: (note exercise, illness, stress, special foods, or other factors that may affect your numbers.)

	Before	After
LUNCH		

COMMENTS: (note exercise, illness, stress, special foods, or other factors that may affect your numbers.)

	Before	After
DINNER		

COMMENTS: (note exercise, illness, stress, special foods, or other factors that may affect your numbers.)

	Before	After
NIGHT		

COMMENTS: (note exercise, illness, stress, special foods, or other factors that may affect your numbers.)

	Before	After
OTHER		

COMMENTS: (note exercise, illness, stress, special foods, or other factors that may affect your numbers.)

	Before	After
OTHER		

COMMENTS: (note exercise, illness, stress, special foods, or other factors that may affect your numbers.)

Date: ____________________

	Before	After
BREAKFAST		

COMMENTS: (note exercise, illness, stress, special foods, or other factors that may affect your numbers.)

	Before	After
LUNCH		

COMMENTS: (note exercise, illness, stress, special foods, or other factors that may affect your numbers.)

	Before	After
DINNER		

COMMENTS: (note exercise, illness, stress, special foods, or other factors that may affect your numbers.)

	Before	After
NIGHT		

COMMENTS: (note exercise, illness, stress, special foods, or other factors that may affect your numbers.)

	Before	After
OTHER		

COMMENTS: (note exercise, illness, stress, special foods, or other factors that may affect your numbers.)

	Before	After
OTHER		

COMMENTS: (note exercise, illness, stress, special foods, or other factors that may affect your numbers.)

BLOOD GLUCOSE JOURNAL

Date: ____________________

	Before	After
BREAKFAST		

COMMENTS: (note exercise, illness, stress, special foods, or other factors that may affect your numbers.)

	Before	After
LUNCH		

COMMENTS: (note exercise, illness, stress, special foods, or other factors that may affect your numbers.)

	Before	After
DINNER		

COMMENTS: (note exercise, illness, stress, special foods, or other factors that may affect your numbers.)

	Before	After
NIGHT		

COMMENTS: (note exercise, illness, stress, special foods, or other factors that may affect your numbers.)

	Before	After
OTHER		

COMMENTS: (note exercise, illness, stress, special foods, or other factors that may affect your numbers.)

	Before	After
OTHER		

COMMENTS: (note exercise, illness, stress, special foods, or other factors that may affect your numbers.)

Date: ____________________

	Before	After
BREAKFAST		

COMMENTS: (note exercise, illness, stress, special foods, or other factors that may affect your numbers.)

	Before	After
LUNCH		

COMMENTS: (note exercise, illness, stress, special foods, or other factors that may affect your numbers.)

	Before	After
DINNER		

COMMENTS: (note exercise, illness, stress, special foods, or other factors that may affect your numbers.)

	Before	After
NIGHT		

COMMENTS: (note exercise, illness, stress, special foods, or other factors that may affect your numbers.)

	Before	After
OTHER		

COMMENTS: (note exercise, illness, stress, special foods, or other factors that may affect your numbers.)

	Before	After
OTHER		

COMMENTS: (note exercise, illness, stress, special foods, or other factors that may affect your numbers.)

BLOOD GLUCOSE JOURNAL

Date: ___________________

	Before	After
BREAKFAST		

COMMENTS: (note exercise, illness, stress, special foods, or other factors that may affect your numbers.)

	Before	After
LUNCH		

COMMENTS: (note exercise, illness, stress, special foods, or other factors that may affect your numbers.)

	Before	After
DINNER		

COMMENTS: (note exercise, illness, stress, special foods, or other factors that may affect your numbers.)

	Before	After
NIGHT		

COMMENTS: (note exercise, illness, stress, special foods, or other factors that may affect your numbers.)

	Before	After
OTHER		

COMMENTS: (note exercise, illness, stress, special foods, or other factors that may affect your numbers.)

	Before	After
OTHER		

COMMENTS: (note exercise, illness, stress, special foods, or other factors that may affect your numbers.)

Date: ___________________

	Before	After
BREAKFAST		

COMMENTS: (note exercise, illness, stress, special foods, or other factors that may affect your numbers.)

	Before	After
LUNCH		

COMMENTS: (note exercise, illness, stress, special foods, or other factors that may affect your numbers.)

	Before	After
DINNER		

COMMENTS: (note exercise, illness, stress, special foods, or other factors that may affect your numbers.)

	Before	After
NIGHT		

COMMENTS: (note exercise, illness, stress, special foods, or other factors that may affect your numbers.)

	Before	After
OTHER		

COMMENTS: (note exercise, illness, stress, special foods, or other factors that may affect your numbers.)

	Before	After
OTHER		

COMMENTS: (note exercise, illness, stress, special foods, or other factors that may affect your numbers.)

BLOOD GLUCOSE JOURNAL

Date: ____________________

	Before	After
BREAKFAST		

COMMENTS: (note exercise, illness, stress, special foods, or other factors that may affect your numbers.)

	Before	After
LUNCH		

COMMENTS: (note exercise, illness, stress, special foods, or other factors that may affect your numbers.)

	Before	After
DINNER		

COMMENTS: (note exercise, illness, stress, special foods, or other factors that may affect your numbers.)

	Before	After
NIGHT		

COMMENTS: (note exercise, illness, stress, special foods, or other factors that may affect your numbers.)

	Before	After
OTHER		

COMMENTS: (note exercise, illness, stress, special foods, or other factors that may affect your numbers.)

	Before	After
OTHER		

COMMENTS: (note exercise, illness, stress, special foods, or other factors that may affect your numbers.)

Date: ____________________

	Before	After
BREAKFAST		

COMMENTS: (note exercise, illness, stress, special foods, or other factors that may affect your numbers.)

	Before	After
LUNCH		

COMMENTS: (note exercise, illness, stress, special foods, or other factors that may affect your numbers.)

	Before	After
DINNER		

COMMENTS: (note exercise, illness, stress, special foods, or other factors that may affect your numbers.)

	Before	After
NIGHT		

COMMENTS: (note exercise, illness, stress, special foods, or other factors that may affect your numbers.)

	Before	After
OTHER		

COMMENTS: (note exercise, illness, stress, special foods, or other factors that may affect your numbers.)

	Before	After
OTHER		

COMMENTS: (note exercise, illness, stress, special foods, or other factors that may affect your numbers.)

BLOOD GLUCOSE JOURNAL

Date: ____________________

	Before	After
BREAKFAST		

COMMENTS: (note exercise, illness, stress, special foods, or other factors that may affect your numbers.)

	Before	After
LUNCH		

COMMENTS: (note exercise, illness, stress, special foods, or other factors that may affect your numbers.)

	Before	After
DINNER		

COMMENTS: (note exercise, illness, stress, special foods, or other factors that may affect your numbers.)

	Before	After
NIGHT		

COMMENTS: (note exercise, illness, stress, special foods, or other factors that may affect your numbers.)

	Before	After
OTHER		

COMMENTS: (note exercise, illness, stress, special foods, or other factors that may affect your numbers.)

	Before	After
OTHER		

COMMENTS: (note exercise, illness, stress, special foods, or other factors that may affect your numbers.)

Date: ____________________

	Before	After
BREAKFAST		

COMMENTS: (note exercise, illness, stress, special foods, or other factors that may affect your numbers.)

	Before	After
LUNCH		

COMMENTS: (note exercise, illness, stress, special foods, or other factors that may affect your numbers.)

	Before	After
DINNER		

COMMENTS: (note exercise, illness, stress, special foods, or other factors that may affect your numbers.)

	Before	After
NIGHT		

COMMENTS: (note exercise, illness, stress, special foods, or other factors that may affect your numbers.)

	Before	After
OTHER		

COMMENTS: (note exercise, illness, stress, special foods, or other factors that may affect your numbers.)

	Before	After
OTHER		

COMMENTS: (note exercise, illness, stress, special foods, or other factors that may affect your numbers.)

BLOOD GLUCOSE JOURNAL

Date: ___________________

	Before	After
BREAKFAST		

COMMENTS: (note exercise, illness, stress, special foods, or other factors that may affect your numbers.)

	Before	After
LUNCH		

COMMENTS: (note exercise, illness, stress, special foods, or other factors that may affect your numbers.)

	Before	After
DINNER		

COMMENTS: (note exercise, illness, stress, special foods, or other factors that may affect your numbers.)

	Before	After
NIGHT		

COMMENTS: (note exercise, illness, stress, special foods, or other factors that may affect your numbers.)

	Before	After
OTHER		

COMMENTS: (note exercise, illness, stress, special foods, or other factors that may affect your numbers.)

	Before	After
OTHER		

COMMENTS: (note exercise, illness, stress, special foods, or other factors that may affect your numbers.)

Date: ____________________

	Before	After
BREAKFAST		

COMMENTS: (note exercise, illness, stress, special foods, or other factors that may affect your numbers.)

	Before	After
LUNCH		

COMMENTS: (note exercise, illness, stress, special foods, or other factors that may affect your numbers.)

	Before	After
DINNER		

COMMENTS: (note exercise, illness, stress, special foods, or other factors that may affect your numbers.)

	Before	After
NIGHT		

COMMENTS: (note exercise, illness, stress, special foods, or other factors that may affect your numbers.)

	Before	After
OTHER		

COMMENTS: (note exercise, illness, stress, special foods, or other factors that may affect your numbers.)

	Before	After
OTHER		

COMMENTS: (note exercise, illness, stress, special foods, or other factors that may affect your numbers.)

BLOOD GLUCOSE JOURNAL

Date: ____________________

	Before	After
BREAKFAST		

COMMENTS: (note exercise, illness, stress, special foods, or other factors that may affect your numbers.)

	Before	After
LUNCH		

COMMENTS: (note exercise, illness, stress, special foods, or other factors that may affect your numbers.)

	Before	After
DINNER		

COMMENTS: (note exercise, illness, stress, special foods, or other factors that may affect your numbers.)

	Before	After
NIGHT		

COMMENTS: (note exercise, illness, stress, special foods, or other factors that may affect your numbers.)

	Before	After
OTHER		

COMMENTS: (note exercise, illness, stress, special foods, or other factors that may affect your numbers.)

	Before	After
OTHER		

COMMENTS: (note exercise, illness, stress, special foods, or other factors that may affect your numbers.)

Date: ____________________

	Before	After
BREAKFAST		

COMMENTS: (note exercise, illness, stress, special foods, or other factors that may affect your numbers.)

	Before	After
LUNCH		

COMMENTS: (note exercise, illness, stress, special foods, or other factors that may affect your numbers.)

	Before	After
DINNER		

COMMENTS: (note exercise, illness, stress, special foods, or other factors that may affect your numbers.)

	Before	After
NIGHT		

COMMENTS: (note exercise, illness, stress, special foods, or other factors that may affect your numbers.)

	Before	After
OTHER		

COMMENTS: (note exercise, illness, stress, special foods, or other factors that may affect your numbers.)

	Before	After
OTHER		

COMMENTS: (note exercise, illness, stress, special foods, or other factors that may affect your numbers.)

BLOOD GLUCOSE JOURNAL

Date: ___________________

	Before	After
BREAKFAST		

COMMENTS: (note exercise, illness, stress, special foods, or other factors that may affect your numbers.)

	Before	After
LUNCH		

COMMENTS: (note exercise, illness, stress, special foods, or other factors that may affect your numbers.)

	Before	After
DINNER		

COMMENTS: (note exercise, illness, stress, special foods, or other factors that may affect your numbers.)

	Before	After
NIGHT		

COMMENTS: (note exercise, illness, stress, special foods, or other factors that may affect your numbers.)

	Before	After
OTHER		

COMMENTS: (note exercise, illness, stress, special foods, or other factors that may affect your numbers.)

	Before	After
OTHER		

COMMENTS: (note exercise, illness, stress, special foods, or other factors that may affect your numbers.)

Date: ____________________

	Before	After
BREAKFAST		

COMMENTS: (note exercise, illness, stress, special foods, or other factors that may affect your numbers.)

	Before	After
LUNCH		

COMMENTS: (note exercise, illness, stress, special foods, or other factors that may affect your numbers.)

	Before	After
DINNER		

COMMENTS: (note exercise, illness, stress, special foods, or other factors that may affect your numbers.)

	Before	After
NIGHT		

COMMENTS: (note exercise, illness, stress, special foods, or other factors that may affect your numbers.)

	Before	After
OTHER		

COMMENTS: (note exercise, illness, stress, special foods, or other factors that may affect your numbers.)

	Before	After
OTHER		

COMMENTS: (note exercise, illness, stress, special foods, or other factors that may affect your numbers.)

BLOOD GLUCOSE JOURNAL

Date: ____________________

	Before	After
BREAKFAST		

COMMENTS: (note exercise, illness, stress, special foods, or other factors that may affect your numbers.)

	Before	After
LUNCH		

COMMENTS: (note exercise, illness, stress, special foods, or other factors that may affect your numbers.)

	Before	After
DINNER		

COMMENTS: (note exercise, illness, stress, special foods, or other factors that may affect your numbers.)

	Before	After
NIGHT		

COMMENTS: (note exercise, illness, stress, special foods, or other factors that may affect your numbers.)

	Before	After
OTHER		

COMMENTS: (note exercise, illness, stress, special foods, or other factors that may affect your numbers.)

	Before	After
OTHER		

COMMENTS: (note exercise, illness, stress, special foods, or other factors that may affect your numbers.)

Date: ____________________

	Before	After
BREAKFAST		

COMMENTS: (note exercise, illness, stress, special foods, or other factors that may affect your numbers.)

	Before	After
LUNCH		

COMMENTS: (note exercise, illness, stress, special foods, or other factors that may affect your numbers.)

	Before	After
DINNER		

COMMENTS: (note exercise, illness, stress, special foods, or other factors that may affect your numbers.)

	Before	After
NIGHT		

COMMENTS: (note exercise, illness, stress, special foods, or other factors that may affect your numbers.)

	Before	After
OTHER		

COMMENTS: (note exercise, illness, stress, special foods, or other factors that may affect your numbers.)

	Before	After
OTHER		

COMMENTS: (note exercise, illness, stress, special foods, or other factors that may affect your numbers.)

BLOOD GLUCOSE JOURNAL

Date: ______________________

	Before	After
BREAKFAST		

COMMENTS: (note exercise, illness, stress, special foods, or other factors that may affect your numbers.)

	Before	After
LUNCH		

COMMENTS: (note exercise, illness, stress, special foods, or other factors that may affect your numbers.)

	Before	After
DINNER		

COMMENTS: (note exercise, illness, stress, special foods, or other factors that may affect your numbers.)

	Before	After
NIGHT		

COMMENTS: (note exercise, illness, stress, special foods, or other factors that may affect your numbers.)

	Before	After
OTHER		

COMMENTS: (note exercise, illness, stress, special foods, or other factors that may affect your numbers.)

	Before	After
OTHER		

COMMENTS: (note exercise, illness, stress, special foods, or other factors that may affect your numbers.)

Date: ____________________

	Before	After
BREAKFAST		

COMMENTS: (note exercise, illness, stress, special foods, or other factors that may affect your numbers.)

	Before	After
LUNCH		

COMMENTS: (note exercise, illness, stress, special foods, or other factors that may affect your numbers.)

	Before	After
DINNER		

COMMENTS: (note exercise, illness, stress, special foods, or other factors that may affect your numbers.)

	Before	After
NIGHT		

COMMENTS: (note exercise, illness, stress, special foods, or other factors that may affect your numbers.)

	Before	After
OTHER		

COMMENTS: (note exercise, illness, stress, special foods, or other factors that may affect your numbers.)

	Before	After
OTHER		

COMMENTS: (note exercise, illness, stress, special foods, or other factors that may affect your numbers.)

BLOOD GLUCOSE JOURNAL

Date: ____________________

	Before	After
BREAKFAST		

COMMENTS: (note exercise, illness, stress, special foods, or other factors that may affect your numbers.)

	Before	After
LUNCH		

COMMENTS: (note exercise, illness, stress, special foods, or other factors that may affect your numbers.)

	Before	After
DINNER		

COMMENTS: (note exercise, illness, stress, special foods, or other factors that may affect your numbers.)

	Before	After
NIGHT		

COMMENTS: (note exercise, illness, stress, special foods, or other factors that may affect your numbers.)

	Before	After
OTHER		

COMMENTS: (note exercise, illness, stress, special foods, or other factors that may affect your numbers.)

	Before	After
OTHER		

COMMENTS: (note exercise, illness, stress, special foods, or other factors that may affect your numbers.)

Date: ____________________

	Before	After
BREAKFAST		

COMMENTS: (note exercise, illness, stress, special foods, or other factors that may affect your numbers.)

	Before	After
LUNCH		

COMMENTS: (note exercise, illness, stress, special foods, or other factors that may affect your numbers.)

	Before	After
DINNER		

COMMENTS: (note exercise, illness, stress, special foods, or other factors that may affect your numbers.)

	Before	After
NIGHT		

COMMENTS: (note exercise, illness, stress, special foods, or other factors that may affect your numbers.)

	Before	After
OTHER		

COMMENTS: (note exercise, illness, stress, special foods, or other factors that may affect your numbers.)

	Before	After
OTHER		

COMMENTS: (note exercise, illness, stress, special foods, or other factors that may affect your numbers.)

BLOOD GLUCOSE JOURNAL

Date: ____________________

	Before	After
BREAKFAST		

COMMENTS: (note exercise, illness, stress, special foods, or other factors that may affect your numbers.)

	Before	After
LUNCH		

COMMENTS: (note exercise, illness, stress, special foods, or other factors that may affect your numbers.)

	Before	After
DINNER		

COMMENTS: (note exercise, illness, stress, special foods, or other factors that may affect your numbers.)

	Before	After
NIGHT		

COMMENTS: (note exercise, illness, stress, special foods, or other factors that may affect your numbers.)

	Before	After
OTHER		

COMMENTS: (note exercise, illness, stress, special foods, or other factors that may affect your numbers.)

	Before	After
OTHER		

COMMENTS: (note exercise, illness, stress, special foods, or other factors that may affect your numbers.)

Date: ____________________

	Before	After
BREAKFAST		

COMMENTS: (note exercise, illness, stress, special foods, or other factors that may affect your numbers.)

	Before	After
LUNCH		

COMMENTS: (note exercise, illness, stress, special foods, or other factors that may affect your numbers.)

	Before	After
DINNER		

COMMENTS: (note exercise, illness, stress, special foods, or other factors that may affect your numbers.)

	Before	After
NIGHT		

COMMENTS: (note exercise, illness, stress, special foods, or other factors that may affect your numbers.)

	Before	After
OTHER		

COMMENTS: (note exercise, illness, stress, special foods, or other factors that may affect your numbers.)

	Before	After
OTHER		

COMMENTS: (note exercise, illness, stress, special foods, or other factors that may affect your numbers.)

BLOOD GLUCOSE JOURNAL

Date: ____________________

	Before	After
BREAKFAST		

COMMENTS: (note exercise, illness, stress, special foods, or other factors that may affect your numbers.)

	Before	After
LUNCH		

COMMENTS: (note exercise, illness, stress, special foods, or other factors that may affect your numbers.)

	Before	After
DINNER		

COMMENTS: (note exercise, illness, stress, special foods, or other factors that may affect your numbers.)

	Before	After
NIGHT		

COMMENTS: (note exercise, illness, stress, special foods, or other factors that may affect your numbers.)

	Before	After
OTHER		

COMMENTS: (note exercise, illness, stress, special foods, or other factors that may affect your numbers.)

	Before	After
OTHER		

COMMENTS: (note exercise, illness, stress, special foods, or other factors that may affect your numbers.)

Date: ________________

	Before	After
BREAKFAST		

COMMENTS: (note exercise, illness, stress, special foods, or other factors that may affect your numbers.)

	Before	After
LUNCH		

COMMENTS: (note exercise, illness, stress, special foods, or other factors that may affect your numbers.)

	Before	After
DINNER		

COMMENTS: (note exercise, illness, stress, special foods, or other factors that may affect your numbers.)

	Before	After
NIGHT		

COMMENTS: (note exercise, illness, stress, special foods, or other factors that may affect your numbers.)

	Before	After
OTHER		

COMMENTS: (note exercise, illness, stress, special foods, or other factors that may affect your numbers.)

	Before	After
OTHER		

COMMENTS: (note exercise, illness, stress, special foods, or other factors that may affect your numbers.)

BLOOD GLUCOSE JOURNAL

Date: ___________________

	Before	After
BREAKFAST		

COMMENTS: (note exercise, illness, stress, special foods, or other factors that may affect your numbers.)

	Before	After
LUNCH		

COMMENTS: (note exercise, illness, stress, special foods, or other factors that may affect your numbers.)

	Before	After
DINNER		

COMMENTS: (note exercise, illness, stress, special foods, or other factors that may affect your numbers.)

	Before	After
NIGHT		

COMMENTS: (note exercise, illness, stress, special foods, or other factors that may affect your numbers.)

	Before	After
OTHER		

COMMENTS: (note exercise, illness, stress, special foods, or other factors that may affect your numbers.)

	Before	After
OTHER		

COMMENTS: (note exercise, illness, stress, special foods, or other factors that may affect your numbers.)

Date: ____________________

	Before	After
BREAKFAST		

COMMENTS: (note exercise, illness, stress, special foods, or other factors that may affect your numbers.)

	Before	After
LUNCH		

COMMENTS: (note exercise, illness, stress, special foods, or other factors that may affect your numbers.)

	Before	After
DINNER		

COMMENTS: (note exercise, illness, stress, special foods, or other factors that may affect your numbers.)

	Before	After
NIGHT		

COMMENTS: (note exercise, illness, stress, special foods, or other factors that may affect your numbers.)

	Before	After
OTHER		

COMMENTS: (note exercise, illness, stress, special foods, or other factors that may affect your numbers.)

	Before	After
OTHER		

COMMENTS: (note exercise, illness, stress, special foods, or other factors that may affect your numbers.)

BLOOD GLUCOSE JOURNAL

Date: ____________________

	Before	After
BREAKFAST		

COMMENTS: (note exercise, illness, stress, special foods, or other factors that may affect your numbers.)

	Before	After
LUNCH		

COMMENTS: (note exercise, illness, stress, special foods, or other factors that may affect your numbers.)

	Before	After
DINNER		

COMMENTS: (note exercise, illness, stress, special foods, or other factors that may affect your numbers.)

	Before	After
NIGHT		

COMMENTS: (note exercise, illness, stress, special foods, or other factors that may affect your numbers.)

	Before	After
OTHER		

COMMENTS: (note exercise, illness, stress, special foods, or other factors that may affect your numbers.)

	Before	After
OTHER		

COMMENTS: (note exercise, illness, stress, special foods, or other factors that may affect your numbers.)

Date: ____________________

	Before	After
BREAKFAST		

COMMENTS: (note exercise, illness, stress, special foods, or other factors that may affect your numbers.)

	Before	After
LUNCH		

COMMENTS: (note exercise, illness, stress, special foods, or other factors that may affect your numbers.)

	Before	After
DINNER		

COMMENTS: (note exercise, illness, stress, special foods, or other factors that may affect your numbers.)

	Before	After
NIGHT		

COMMENTS: (note exercise, illness, stress, special foods, or other factors that may affect your numbers.)

	Before	After
OTHER		

COMMENTS: (note exercise, illness, stress, special foods, or other factors that may affect your numbers.)

	Before	After
OTHER		

COMMENTS: (note exercise, illness, stress, special foods, or other factors that may affect your numbers.)

BLOOD GLUCOSE JOURNAL

Date: ____________________

	Before	After
BREAKFAST		

COMMENTS: (note exercise, illness, stress, special foods, or other factors that may affect your numbers.)

	Before	After
LUNCH		

COMMENTS: (note exercise, illness, stress, special foods, or other factors that may affect your numbers.)

	Before	After
DINNER		

COMMENTS: (note exercise, illness, stress, special foods, or other factors that may affect your numbers.)

	Before	After
NIGHT		

COMMENTS: (note exercise, illness, stress, special foods, or other factors that may affect your numbers.)

	Before	After
OTHER		

COMMENTS: (note exercise, illness, stress, special foods, or other factors that may affect your numbers.)

	Before	After
OTHER		

COMMENTS: (note exercise, illness, stress, special foods, or other factors that may affect your numbers.)

Date: ____________________

	Before	After
BREAKFAST		

COMMENTS: (note exercise, illness, stress, special foods, or other factors that may affect your numbers.)

	Before	After
LUNCH		

COMMENTS: (note exercise, illness, stress, special foods, or other factors that may affect your numbers.)

	Before	After
DINNER		

COMMENTS: (note exercise, illness, stress, special foods, or other factors that may affect your numbers.)

	Before	After
NIGHT		

COMMENTS: (note exercise, illness, stress, special foods, or other factors that may affect your numbers.)

	Before	After
OTHER		

COMMENTS: (note exercise, illness, stress, special foods, or other factors that may affect your numbers.)

	Before	After
OTHER		

COMMENTS: (note exercise, illness, stress, special foods, or other factors that may affect your numbers.)

BLOOD GLUCOSE JOURNAL

Date: ____________________

	Before	After
BREAKFAST		

COMMENTS: (note exercise, illness, stress, special foods, or other factors that may affect your numbers.)

	Before	After
LUNCH		

COMMENTS: (note exercise, illness, stress, special foods, or other factors that may affect your numbers.)

	Before	After
DINNER		

COMMENTS: (note exercise, illness, stress, special foods, or other factors that may affect your numbers.)

	Before	After
NIGHT		

COMMENTS: (note exercise, illness, stress, special foods, or other factors that may affect your numbers.)

	Before	After
OTHER		

COMMENTS: (note exercise, illness, stress, special foods, or other factors that may affect your numbers.)

	Before	After
OTHER		

COMMENTS: (note exercise, illness, stress, special foods, or other factors that may affect your numbers.)

Date: ____________________

	Before	After
BREAKFAST		

COMMENTS: (note exercise, illness, stress, special foods, or other factors that may affect your numbers.)

	Before	After
LUNCH		

COMMENTS: (note exercise, illness, stress, special foods, or other factors that may affect your numbers.)

	Before	After
DINNER		

COMMENTS: (note exercise, illness, stress, special foods, or other factors that may affect your numbers.)

	Before	After
NIGHT		

COMMENTS: (note exercise, illness, stress, special foods, or other factors that may affect your numbers.)

	Before	After
OTHER		

COMMENTS: (note exercise, illness, stress, special foods, or other factors that may affect your numbers.)

	Before	After
OTHER		

COMMENTS: (note exercise, illness, stress, special foods, or other factors that may affect your numbers.)

Date: ________________

	Before	After
BREAKFAST		

COMMENTS: (note exercise, illness, stress, special foods, or other factors that may affect your numbers.)

	Before	After
LUNCH		

COMMENTS: (note exercise, illness, stress, special foods, or other factors that may affect your numbers.)

	Before	After
DINNER		

COMMENTS: (note exercise, illness, stress, special foods, or other factors that may affect your numbers.)

	Before	After
NIGHT		

COMMENTS: (note exercise, illness, stress, special foods, or other factors that may affect your numbers.)

	Before	After
OTHER		

COMMENTS: (note exercise, illness, stress, special foods, or other factors that may affect your numbers.)

	Before	After
OTHER		

COMMENTS: (note exercise, illness, stress, special foods, or other factors that may affect your numbers.)

Date: ___________________

	Before	After
BREAKFAST		

COMMENTS: (note exercise, illness, stress, special foods, or other factors that may affect your numbers.)

	Before	After
LUNCH		

COMMENTS: (note exercise, illness, stress, special foods, or other factors that may affect your numbers.)

	Before	After
DINNER		

COMMENTS: (note exercise, illness, stress, special foods, or other factors that may affect your numbers.)

	Before	After
NIGHT		

COMMENTS: (note exercise, illness, stress, special foods, or other factors that may affect your numbers.)

	Before	After
OTHER		

COMMENTS: (note exercise, illness, stress, special foods, or other factors that may affect your numbers.)

	Before	After
OTHER		

COMMENTS: (note exercise, illness, stress, special foods, or other factors that may affect your numbers.)

BLOOD GLUCOSE JOURNAL

Date: ____________________

	Before	After
BREAKFAST		

COMMENTS: (note exercise, illness, stress, special foods, or other factors that may affect your numbers.)

	Before	After
LUNCH		

COMMENTS: (note exercise, illness, stress, special foods, or other factors that may affect your numbers.)

	Before	After
DINNER		

COMMENTS: (note exercise, illness, stress, special foods, or other factors that may affect your numbers.)

	Before	After
NIGHT		

COMMENTS: (note exercise, illness, stress, special foods, or other factors that may affect your numbers.)

	Before	After
OTHER		

COMMENTS: (note exercise, illness, stress, special foods, or other factors that may affect your numbers.)

	Before	After
OTHER		

COMMENTS: (note exercise, illness, stress, special foods, or other factors that may affect your numbers.)

Date: ________________

	Before	After
BREAKFAST		

COMMENTS: (note exercise, illness, stress, special foods, or other factors that may affect your numbers.)

	Before	After
LUNCH		

COMMENTS: (note exercise, illness, stress, special foods, or other factors that may affect your numbers.)

	Before	After
DINNER		

COMMENTS: (note exercise, illness, stress, special foods, or other factors that may affect your numbers.)

	Before	After
NIGHT		

COMMENTS: (note exercise, illness, stress, special foods, or other factors that may affect your numbers.)

	Before	After
OTHER		

COMMENTS: (note exercise, illness, stress, special foods, or other factors that may affect your numbers.)

	Before	After
OTHER		

COMMENTS: (note exercise, illness, stress, special foods, or other factors that may affect your numbers.)

BLOOD GLUCOSE JOURNAL

Date: ___________________

	Before	After
BREAKFAST		

COMMENTS: (note exercise, illness, stress, special foods, or other factors that may affect your numbers.)

	Before	After
LUNCH		

COMMENTS: (note exercise, illness, stress, special foods, or other factors that may affect your numbers.)

	Before	After
DINNER		

COMMENTS: (note exercise, illness, stress, special foods, or other factors that may affect your numbers.)

	Before	After
NIGHT		

COMMENTS: (note exercise, illness, stress, special foods, or other factors that may affect your numbers.)

	Before	After
OTHER		

COMMENTS: (note exercise, illness, stress, special foods, or other factors that may affect your numbers.)

	Before	After
OTHER		

COMMENTS: (note exercise, illness, stress, special foods, or other factors that may affect your numbers.)

Date: ____________________

	Before	After
BREAKFAST		

COMMENTS: (note exercise, illness, stress, special foods, or other factors that may affect your numbers.)

	Before	After
LUNCH		

COMMENTS: (note exercise, illness, stress, special foods, or other factors that may affect your numbers.)

	Before	After
DINNER		

COMMENTS: (note exercise, illness, stress, special foods, or other factors that may affect your numbers.)

	Before	After
NIGHT		

COMMENTS: (note exercise, illness, stress, special foods, or other factors that may affect your numbers.)

	Before	After
OTHER		

COMMENTS: (note exercise, illness, stress, special foods, or other factors that may affect your numbers.)

	Before	After
OTHER		

COMMENTS: (note exercise, illness, stress, special foods, or other factors that may affect your numbers.)

BLOOD GLUCOSE JOURNAL

Date: ____________________

	Before	After
BREAKFAST		

COMMENTS: (note exercise, illness, stress, special foods, or other factors that may affect your numbers.)

	Before	After
LUNCH		

COMMENTS: (note exercise, illness, stress, special foods, or other factors that may affect your numbers.)

	Before	After
DINNER		

COMMENTS: (note exercise, illness, stress, special foods, or other factors that may affect your numbers.)

	Before	After
NIGHT		

COMMENTS: (note exercise, illness, stress, special foods, or other factors that may affect your numbers.)

	Before	After
OTHER		

COMMENTS: (note exercise, illness, stress, special foods, or other factors that may affect your numbers.)

	Before	After
OTHER		

COMMENTS: (note exercise, illness, stress, special foods, or other factors that may affect your numbers.)

Date: ___________________

	Before	After
BREAKFAST		

COMMENTS: (note exercise, illness, stress, special foods, or other factors that may affect your numbers.)

	Before	After
LUNCH		

COMMENTS: (note exercise, illness, stress, special foods, or other factors that may affect your numbers.)

	Before	After
DINNER		

COMMENTS: (note exercise, illness, stress, special foods, or other factors that may affect your numbers.)

	Before	After
NIGHT		

COMMENTS: (note exercise, illness, stress, special foods, or other factors that may affect your numbers.)

	Before	After
OTHER		

COMMENTS: (note exercise, illness, stress, special foods, or other factors that may affect your numbers.)

	Before	After
OTHER		

COMMENTS: (note exercise, illness, stress, special foods, or other factors that may affect your numbers.)

BLOOD GLUCOSE JOURNAL

Date: ____________________

	Before	After
BREAKFAST		

COMMENTS: (note exercise, illness, stress, special foods, or other factors that may affect your numbers.)

	Before	After
LUNCH		

COMMENTS: (note exercise, illness, stress, special foods, or other factors that may affect your numbers.)

	Before	After
DINNER		

COMMENTS: (note exercise, illness, stress, special foods, or other factors that may affect your numbers.)

	Before	After
NIGHT		

COMMENTS: (note exercise, illness, stress, special foods, or other factors that may affect your numbers.)

	Before	After
OTHER		

COMMENTS: (note exercise, illness, stress, special foods, or other factors that may affect your numbers.)

	Before	After
OTHER		

COMMENTS: (note exercise, illness, stress, special foods, or other factors that may affect your numbers.)

Date: ____________________

	Before	After
BREAKFAST		

COMMENTS: (note exercise, illness, stress, special foods, or other factors that may affect your numbers.)

	Before	After
LUNCH		

COMMENTS: (note exercise, illness, stress, special foods, or other factors that may affect your numbers.)

	Before	After
DINNER		

COMMENTS: (note exercise, illness, stress, special foods, or other factors that may affect your numbers.)

	Before	After
NIGHT		

COMMENTS: (note exercise, illness, stress, special foods, or other factors that may affect your numbers.)

	Before	After
OTHER		

COMMENTS: (note exercise, illness, stress, special foods, or other factors that may affect your numbers.)

	Before	After
OTHER		

COMMENTS: (note exercise, illness, stress, special foods, or other factors that may affect your numbers.)

BLOOD GLUCOSE JOURNAL

Date: ____________________

	Before	After
BREAKFAST		

COMMENTS: (note exercise, illness, stress, special foods, or other factors that may affect your numbers.)

	Before	After
LUNCH		

COMMENTS: (note exercise, illness, stress, special foods, or other factors that may affect your numbers.)

	Before	After
DINNER		

COMMENTS: (note exercise, illness, stress, special foods, or other factors that may affect your numbers.)

	Before	After
NIGHT		

COMMENTS: (note exercise, illness, stress, special foods, or other factors that may affect your numbers.)

	Before	After
OTHER		

COMMENTS: (note exercise, illness, stress, special foods, or other factors that may affect your numbers.)

	Before	After
OTHER		

COMMENTS: (note exercise, illness, stress, special foods, or other factors that may affect your numbers.)

Date: ____________________

	Before	After
BREAKFAST		

COMMENTS: (note exercise, illness, stress, special foods, or other factors that may affect your numbers.)

	Before	After
LUNCH		

COMMENTS: (note exercise, illness, stress, special foods, or other factors that may affect your numbers.)

	Before	After
DINNER		

COMMENTS: (note exercise, illness, stress, special foods, or other factors that may affect your numbers.)

	Before	After
NIGHT		

COMMENTS: (note exercise, illness, stress, special foods, or other factors that may affect your numbers.)

	Before	After
OTHER		

COMMENTS: (note exercise, illness, stress, special foods, or other factors that may affect your numbers.)

	Before	After
OTHER		

COMMENTS: (note exercise, illness, stress, special foods, or other factors that may affect your numbers.)

BLOOD GLUCOSE JOURNAL

Date: ____________________

	Before	After
BREAKFAST		

COMMENTS: (note exercise, illness, stress, special foods, or other factors that may affect your numbers.)

	Before	After
LUNCH		

COMMENTS: (note exercise, illness, stress, special foods, or other factors that may affect your numbers.)

	Before	After
DINNER		

COMMENTS: (note exercise, illness, stress, special foods, or other factors that may affect your numbers.)

	Before	After
NIGHT		

COMMENTS: (note exercise, illness, stress, special foods, or other factors that may affect your numbers.)

	Before	After
OTHER		

COMMENTS: (note exercise, illness, stress, special foods, or other factors that may affect your numbers.)

	Before	After
OTHER		

COMMENTS: (note exercise, illness, stress, special foods, or other factors that may affect your numbers.)

Date: ____________________

	Before	After
BREAKFAST		

COMMENTS: (note exercise, illness, stress, special foods, or other factors that may affect your numbers.)

	Before	After
LUNCH		

COMMENTS: (note exercise, illness, stress, special foods, or other factors that may affect your numbers.)

	Before	After
DINNER		

COMMENTS: (note exercise, illness, stress, special foods, or other factors that may affect your numbers.)

	Before	After
NIGHT		

COMMENTS: (note exercise, illness, stress, special foods, or other factors that may affect your numbers.)

	Before	After
OTHER		

COMMENTS: (note exercise, illness, stress, special foods, or other factors that may affect your numbers.)

	Before	After
OTHER		

COMMENTS: (note exercise, illness, stress, special foods, or other factors that may affect your numbers.)

BLOOD GLUCOSE JOURNAL

Date: ___________________

	Before	After
BREAKFAST		

COMMENTS: (note exercise, illness, stress, special foods, or other factors that may affect your numbers.)

	Before	After
LUNCH		

COMMENTS: (note exercise, illness, stress, special foods, or other factors that may affect your numbers.)

	Before	After
DINNER		

COMMENTS: (note exercise, illness, stress, special foods, or other factors that may affect your numbers.)

	Before	After
NIGHT		

COMMENTS: (note exercise, illness, stress, special foods, or other factors that may affect your numbers.)

	Before	After
OTHER		

COMMENTS: (note exercise, illness, stress, special foods, or other factors that may affect your numbers.)

	Before	After
OTHER		

COMMENTS: (note exercise, illness, stress, special foods, or other factors that may affect your numbers.)

Date: ____________________

	Before	After
BREAKFAST		

COMMENTS: (note exercise, illness, stress, special foods, or other factors that may affect your numbers.)

	Before	After
LUNCH		

COMMENTS: (note exercise, illness, stress, special foods, or other factors that may affect your numbers.)

	Before	After
DINNER		

COMMENTS: (note exercise, illness, stress, special foods, or other factors that may affect your numbers.)

	Before	After
NIGHT		

COMMENTS: (note exercise, illness, stress, special foods, or other factors that may affect your numbers.)

	Before	After
OTHER		

COMMENTS: (note exercise, illness, stress, special foods, or other factors that may affect your numbers.)

	Before	After
OTHER		

COMMENTS: (note exercise, illness, stress, special foods, or other factors that may affect your numbers.)

BLOOD GLUCOSE JOURNAL

Date: ____________________

	Before	After
BREAKFAST		

COMMENTS: (note exercise, illness, stress, special foods, or other factors that may affect your numbers.)

	Before	After
LUNCH		

COMMENTS: (note exercise, illness, stress, special foods, or other factors that may affect your numbers.)

	Before	After
DINNER		

COMMENTS: (note exercise, illness, stress, special foods, or other factors that may affect your numbers.)

	Before	After
NIGHT		

COMMENTS: (note exercise, illness, stress, special foods, or other factors that may affect your numbers.)

	Before	After
OTHER		

COMMENTS: (note exercise, illness, stress, special foods, or other factors that may affect your numbers.)

	Before	After
OTHER		

COMMENTS: (note exercise, illness, stress, special foods, or other factors that may affect your numbers.)

Date: ___________________

	Before	After
BREAKFAST		

COMMENTS: (note exercise, illness, stress, special foods, or other factors that may affect your numbers.)

	Before	After
LUNCH		

COMMENTS: (note exercise, illness, stress, special foods, or other factors that may affect your numbers.)

	Before	After
DINNER		

COMMENTS: (note exercise, illness, stress, special foods, or other factors that may affect your numbers.)

	Before	After
NIGHT		

COMMENTS: (note exercise, illness, stress, special foods, or other factors that may affect your numbers.)

	Before	After
OTHER		

COMMENTS: (note exercise, illness, stress, special foods, or other factors that may affect your numbers.)

	Before	After
OTHER		

COMMENTS: (note exercise, illness, stress, special foods, or other factors that may affect your numbers.)

BLOOD GLUCOSE JOURNAL

Date: ____________________

	Before	After
BREAKFAST		

COMMENTS: (note exercise, illness, stress, special foods, or other factors that may affect your numbers.)

	Before	After
LUNCH		

COMMENTS: (note exercise, illness, stress, special foods, or other factors that may affect your numbers.)

	Before	After
DINNER		

COMMENTS: (note exercise, illness, stress, special foods, or other factors that may affect your numbers.)

	Before	After
NIGHT		

COMMENTS: (note exercise, illness, stress, special foods, or other factors that may affect your numbers.)

	Before	After
OTHER		

COMMENTS: (note exercise, illness, stress, special foods, or other factors that may affect your numbers.)

	Before	After
OTHER		

COMMENTS: (note exercise, illness, stress, special foods, or other factors that may affect your numbers.)

Date: ____________________

	Before	After
BREAKFAST		

COMMENTS: (note exercise, illness, stress, special foods, or other factors that may affect your numbers.)

	Before	After
LUNCH		

COMMENTS: (note exercise, illness, stress, special foods, or other factors that may affect your numbers.)

	Before	After
DINNER		

COMMENTS: (note exercise, illness, stress, special foods, or other factors that may affect your numbers.)

	Before	After
NIGHT		

COMMENTS: (note exercise, illness, stress, special foods, or other factors that may affect your numbers.)

	Before	After
OTHER		

COMMENTS: (note exercise, illness, stress, special foods, or other factors that may affect your numbers.)

	Before	After
OTHER		

COMMENTS: (note exercise, illness, stress, special foods, or other factors that may affect your numbers.)

BLOOD GLUCOSE JOURNAL

Date: ____________________

	Before	After
BREAKFAST		

COMMENTS: (note exercise, illness, stress, special foods, or other factors that may affect your numbers.)

	Before	After
LUNCH		

COMMENTS: (note exercise, illness, stress, special foods, or other factors that may affect your numbers.)

	Before	After
DINNER		

COMMENTS: (note exercise, illness, stress, special foods, or other factors that may affect your numbers.)

	Before	After
NIGHT		

COMMENTS: (note exercise, illness, stress, special foods, or other factors that may affect your numbers.)

	Before	After
OTHER		

COMMENTS: (note exercise, illness, stress, special foods, or other factors that may affect your numbers.)

	Before	After
OTHER		

COMMENTS: (note exercise, illness, stress, special foods, or other factors that may affect your numbers.)

Date: ____________________

	Before	After
BREAKFAST		

COMMENTS: (note exercise, illness, stress, special foods, or other factors that may affect your numbers.)

	Before	After
LUNCH		

COMMENTS: (note exercise, illness, stress, special foods, or other factors that may affect your numbers.)

	Before	After
DINNER		

COMMENTS: (note exercise, illness, stress, special foods, or other factors that may affect your numbers.)

	Before	After
NIGHT		

COMMENTS: (note exercise, illness, stress, special foods, or other factors that may affect your numbers.)

	Before	After
OTHER		

COMMENTS: (note exercise, illness, stress, special foods, or other factors that may affect your numbers.)

	Before	After
OTHER		

COMMENTS: (note exercise, illness, stress, special foods, or other factors that may affect your numbers.)

BLOOD GLUCOSE JOURNAL

Date: ____________________

	Before	After
BREAKFAST		

COMMENTS: (note exercise, illness, stress, special foods, or other factors that may affect your numbers.)

	Before	After
LUNCH		

COMMENTS: (note exercise, illness, stress, special foods, or other factors that may affect your numbers.)

	Before	After
DINNER		

COMMENTS: (note exercise, illness, stress, special foods, or other factors that may affect your numbers.)

	Before	After
NIGHT		

COMMENTS: (note exercise, illness, stress, special foods, or other factors that may affect your numbers.)

	Before	After
OTHER		

COMMENTS: (note exercise, illness, stress, special foods, or other factors that may affect your numbers.)

	Before	After
OTHER		

COMMENTS: (note exercise, illness, stress, special foods, or other factors that may affect your numbers.)

Date: ____________________

	Before	After
BREAKFAST		

COMMENTS: (note exercise, illness, stress, special foods, or other factors that may affect your numbers.)

	Before	After
LUNCH		

COMMENTS: (note exercise, illness, stress, special foods, or other factors that may affect your numbers.)

	Before	After
DINNER		

COMMENTS: (note exercise, illness, stress, special foods, or other factors that may affect your numbers.)

	Before	After
NIGHT		

COMMENTS: (note exercise, illness, stress, special foods, or other factors that may affect your numbers.)

	Before	After
OTHER		

COMMENTS: (note exercise, illness, stress, special foods, or other factors that may affect your numbers.)

	Before	After
OTHER		

COMMENTS: (note exercise, illness, stress, special foods, or other factors that may affect your numbers.)

BLOOD GLUCOSE JOURNAL

Date: ___________________

	Before	After
BREAKFAST		

COMMENTS: (note exercise, illness, stress, special foods, or other factors that may affect your numbers.)

	Before	After
LUNCH		

COMMENTS: (note exercise, illness, stress, special foods, or other factors that may affect your numbers.)

	Before	After
DINNER		

COMMENTS: (note exercise, illness, stress, special foods, or other factors that may affect your numbers.)

	Before	After
NIGHT		

COMMENTS: (note exercise, illness, stress, special foods, or other factors that may affect your numbers.)

	Before	After
OTHER		

COMMENTS: (note exercise, illness, stress, special foods, or other factors that may affect your numbers.)

	Before	After
OTHER		

COMMENTS: (note exercise, illness, stress, special foods, or other factors that may affect your numbers.)

Date: ____________________

	Before	After
BREAKFAST		

COMMENTS: (note exercise, illness, stress, special foods, or other factors that may affect your numbers.)

	Before	After
LUNCH		

COMMENTS: (note exercise, illness, stress, special foods, or other factors that may affect your numbers.)

	Before	After
DINNER		

COMMENTS: (note exercise, illness, stress, special foods, or other factors that may affect your numbers.)

	Before	After
NIGHT		

COMMENTS: (note exercise, illness, stress, special foods, or other factors that may affect your numbers.)

	Before	After
OTHER		

COMMENTS: (note exercise, illness, stress, special foods, or other factors that may affect your numbers.)

	Before	After
OTHER		

COMMENTS: (note exercise, illness, stress, special foods, or other factors that may affect your numbers.)

BLOOD GLUCOSE JOURNAL

Date: ____________________

	Before	After
BREAKFAST		

COMMENTS: (note exercise, illness, stress, special foods, or other factors that may affect your numbers.)

	Before	After
LUNCH		

COMMENTS: (note exercise, illness, stress, special foods, or other factors that may affect your numbers.)

	Before	After
DINNER		

COMMENTS: (note exercise, illness, stress, special foods, or other factors that may affect your numbers.)

	Before	After
NIGHT		

COMMENTS: (note exercise, illness, stress, special foods, or other factors that may affect your numbers.)

	Before	After
OTHER		

COMMENTS: (note exercise, illness, stress, special foods, or other factors that may affect your numbers.)

	Before	After
OTHER		

COMMENTS: (note exercise, illness, stress, special foods, or other factors that may affect your numbers.)

Date: ____________________

	Before	After
BREAKFAST		

COMMENTS: (note exercise, illness, stress, special foods, or other factors that may affect your numbers.)

	Before	After
LUNCH		

COMMENTS: (note exercise, illness, stress, special foods, or other factors that may affect your numbers.)

	Before	After
DINNER		

COMMENTS: (note exercise, illness, stress, special foods, or other factors that may affect your numbers.)

	Before	After
NIGHT		

COMMENTS: (note exercise, illness, stress, special foods, or other factors that may affect your numbers.)

	Before	After
OTHER		

COMMENTS: (note exercise, illness, stress, special foods, or other factors that may affect your numbers.)

	Before	After
OTHER		

COMMENTS: (note exercise, illness, stress, special foods, or other factors that may affect your numbers.)

BLOOD GLUCOSE JOURNAL

Date: ____________________

	Before	After
BREAKFAST		

COMMENTS: (note exercise, illness, stress, special foods, or other factors that may affect your numbers.)

	Before	After
LUNCH		

COMMENTS: (note exercise, illness, stress, special foods, or other factors that may affect your numbers.)

	Before	After
DINNER		

COMMENTS: (note exercise, illness, stress, special foods, or other factors that may affect your numbers.)

	Before	After
NIGHT		

COMMENTS: (note exercise, illness, stress, special foods, or other factors that may affect your numbers.)

	Before	After
OTHER		

COMMENTS: (note exercise, illness, stress, special foods, or other factors that may affect your numbers.)

	Before	After
OTHER		

COMMENTS: (note exercise, illness, stress, special foods, or other factors that may affect your numbers.)

Date: ___________________

	Before	After
BREAKFAST		

COMMENTS: (note exercise, illness, stress, special foods, or other factors that may affect your numbers.)

	Before	After
LUNCH		

COMMENTS: (note exercise, illness, stress, special foods, or other factors that may affect your numbers.)

	Before	After
DINNER		

COMMENTS: (note exercise, illness, stress, special foods, or other factors that may affect your numbers.)

	Before	After
NIGHT		

COMMENTS: (note exercise, illness, stress, special foods, or other factors that may affect your numbers.)

	Before	After
OTHER		

COMMENTS: (note exercise, illness, stress, special foods, or other factors that may affect your numbers.)

	Before	After
OTHER		

COMMENTS: (note exercise, illness, stress, special foods, or other factors that may affect your numbers.)

BLOOD GLUCOSE JOURNAL

Date: ______________

	Before	After
BREAKFAST		

COMMENTS: (note exercise, illness, stress, special foods, or other factors that may affect your numbers.)

	Before	After
LUNCH		

COMMENTS: (note exercise, illness, stress, special foods, or other factors that may affect your numbers.)

	Before	After
DINNER		

COMMENTS: (note exercise, illness, stress, special foods, or other factors that may affect your numbers.)

	Before	After
NIGHT		

COMMENTS: (note exercise, illness, stress, special foods, or other factors that may affect your numbers.)

	Before	After
OTHER		

COMMENTS: (note exercise, illness, stress, special foods, or other factors that may affect your numbers.)

	Before	After
OTHER		

COMMENTS: (note exercise, illness, stress, special foods, or other factors that may affect your numbers.)

Date: ____________________

	Before	After
BREAKFAST		

COMMENTS: (note exercise, illness, stress, special foods, or other factors that may affect your numbers.)

	Before	After
LUNCH		

COMMENTS: (note exercise, illness, stress, special foods, or other factors that may affect your numbers.)

	Before	After
DINNER		

COMMENTS: (note exercise, illness, stress, special foods, or other factors that may affect your numbers.)

	Before	After
NIGHT		

COMMENTS: (note exercise, illness, stress, special foods, or other factors that may affect your numbers.)

	Before	After
OTHER		

COMMENTS: (note exercise, illness, stress, special foods, or other factors that may affect your numbers.)

	Before	After
OTHER		

COMMENTS: (note exercise, illness, stress, special foods, or other factors that may affect your numbers.)

BLOOD GLUCOSE JOURNAL

Date: ____________________

	Before	After
BREAKFAST		

COMMENTS: (note exercise, illness, stress, special foods, or other factors that may affect your numbers.)

	Before	After
LUNCH		

COMMENTS: (note exercise, illness, stress, special foods, or other factors that may affect your numbers.)

	Before	After
DINNER		

COMMENTS: (note exercise, illness, stress, special foods, or other factors that may affect your numbers.)

	Before	After
NIGHT		

COMMENTS: (note exercise, illness, stress, special foods, or other factors that may affect your numbers.)

	Before	After
OTHER		

COMMENTS: (note exercise, illness, stress, special foods, or other factors that may affect your numbers.)

	Before	After
OTHER		

COMMENTS: (note exercise, illness, stress, special foods, or other factors that may affect your numbers.)

Date: ___________________

	Before	After
BREAKFAST		

COMMENTS: (note exercise, illness, stress, special foods, or other factors that may affect your numbers.)

	Before	After
LUNCH		

COMMENTS: (note exercise, illness, stress, special foods, or other factors that may affect your numbers.)

	Before	After
DINNER		

COMMENTS: (note exercise, illness, stress, special foods, or other factors that may affect your numbers.)

	Before	After
NIGHT		

COMMENTS: (note exercise, illness, stress, special foods, or other factors that may affect your numbers.)

	Before	After
OTHER		

COMMENTS: (note exercise, illness, stress, special foods, or other factors that may affect your numbers.)

	Before	After
OTHER		

COMMENTS: (note exercise, illness, stress, special foods, or other factors that may affect your numbers.)

BLOOD GLUCOSE JOURNAL

Date: ________________

	Before	After
BREAKFAST		

COMMENTS: (note exercise, illness, stress, special foods, or other factors that may affect your numbers.)

	Before	After
LUNCH		

COMMENTS: (note exercise, illness, stress, special foods, or other factors that may affect your numbers.)

	Before	After
DINNER		

COMMENTS: (note exercise, illness, stress, special foods, or other factors that may affect your numbers.)

	Before	After
NIGHT		

COMMENTS: (note exercise, illness, stress, special foods, or other factors that may affect your numbers.)

	Before	After
OTHER		

COMMENTS: (note exercise, illness, stress, special foods, or other factors that may affect your numbers.)

	Before	After
OTHER		

COMMENTS: (note exercise, illness, stress, special foods, or other factors that may affect your numbers.)

NOTES

NOTES

NOTES

NOTES

NOTES

NOTES

ABOUT THE AUTHOR

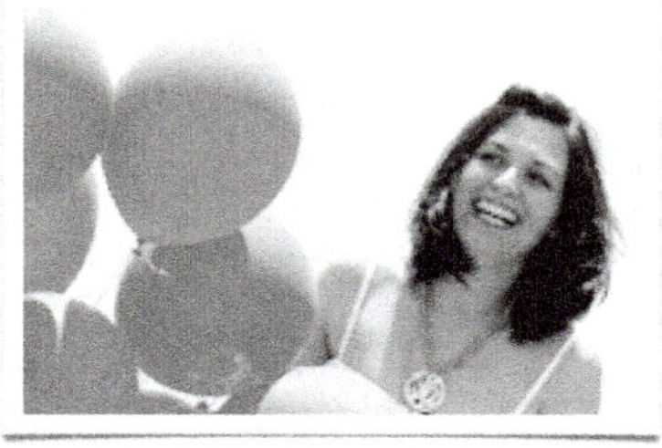

Vivian is an entrepreneur, mentor, speaker, author, and creator of a host of self-help journals, she is known as a tenacious, untiring entrepreneur. Following the success of her book, "Pink Slip to Product Launch in a Weak Economy", and landing her own product line onto the shelves of Whole Foods Markets and 200 retail stores in less than 12 months, Vivian decided to use her business experience and her passion for entrepreneurship to help people build successful businesses. Vivian also created a successful publishing company, and her inspirational journals are now helping thousands of people worldwide record their magical life's moments and helping teach kids and adults the importance of gratitude.

Vivian is passionate about helping people reach their potential! If you'd like to change your health, your financial future and be mentored by her personally, let's chat!

Visit Vivian's website for videos about her journals:
www.viviantenorio.com

Vivian's story has been featured on: CBS The Talk - The Today Show - Good Morning America - Good Morning Texas - Maria Shiver's The Women's Conference - The Willis Report - WomenEntrepreneur.com - Fox Business News - Hybrid Mom - ABC News NOW - Tory Johnson's Spark & Hustle